HOLISTIC FIRST-AID

Healing Emergencies Naturally

by

Dr. Earendil M. Spindelilus D.N.M., M.H., C.R., PSc.D

HOLISTIC FIRST-AID

COPYRIGHT © 2019 BY EARENDIL M. SPINDELILUS

ALL RIGHTS RESERVED.

PUBLISHED BY TREE OF LIFE HOLISTIC WELLNESS CENTER

COVER ART BY EARENDIL AND PEGGY SPINDELILUS

NO PART OF THIS BOOK MAY BE REPRODUCED IN ANY WRITTEN, ELECTRONIC, RECORDING OR PHOTOGRAPHING WITHOUT WRITTEN PERMISSION OF THE PUBLISHER OR AUTHOR.

FIRST EDITION.

ISBN: 9781709456848

DISCLAIMER

THIS BOOK IS INTENDED TO PROVIDE INFORMATION ON THE SUBJECT OF HOLISTIC FIRST AID, THIS INFORMATION PRESENTED IS NOT INTENDED AS A SUBSTITUTE FOR MEDICAL TRAINING OR ADVICE, BUT EVERY EFFORT HAS BEEN MADE TO ENSURE ACCURACY.

THE BOOK IS SOLD WITH THE UNDERSTANDING THAT THE PUBLISHER AND AUTHOR ARE NOT LIABLE FOR ANY MISCONCEPTION OR MISUSE OF THE INFORMATION PROVIDED AND SHALL HAVE NEITHER LIABILITY NOR RESPONSIBILITY TO ANY PERSON OR ENTITY WITH RESPECT TO ANY LOSS, DAMAGE OR INJURY CAUSED OR ALLEGED TO BE CAUSED DIRECTLY OR INDIRECTLY BY THE SAID INFORMATION.

Table of Contents

DEDICATION..5

CHAPTER 1 INTRODUCTION......................................6

CHAPTER 2 BASIC FIRST-AID...................................9

2.1 Burns..9

2.2 Rashes..21

2.3 Bites and Stings...30

2.4 Lice...39

2.5 Warts..41

2.6 Abrasions/bruises..44

CHAPTER 3 INTERMEDIATE FIRST-AID................46

3.1 Ear Infections..46

3.2 Dental..50

3.3 Infections...54

3.4 Allergic Reactions...59

3.5 Bleeding – Minor..65

3.6 Eye Injuries and Infections....................................70

CHAPTER 4 ADVANCED..74

4.1 Major Bleeding/Shock/Deep Cuts and Wounds....74

4.2 Poisoning...81

4.3 Broken Bones..90

4.4 Heart attack/Stroke……………………………………..…94

4.5 Pain Management……………………………………….98

CHAPTER 5 A SAMPLE FIRST-AID KIT……………………106

5.1 First Aid Kit Supplies…………………………………….......106

5.2 How to make your own medications…………………………...109

ABOUT THE AUTHOR……………………………………………...113

DEDICATION

To my wife and best friend Peggy, who has stood beside me and put up with all of my time spent getting one degree or certification after another.

To Waya and Sinde, our furry children who love us unconditionally

I would also like to express my gratitude for all of the patients who have taught me so much about how to be a doctor.

Not all doctors are healers and not all healers are doctors.

CHAPTER 1

Introduction

"An Herbalist in every home and a Master Herbalist in every community"
Dr. John R. Christopher

I can say that while technology seems to have made lives easier, I would not say it has made them better. A case in point is the lack of knowledge these days in the proper care and feeding of emergency situations. There was a time when most folks had at least a rudimentary understanding of first aid care and could handle most situations on their own. Most families or villages had a skilled healer in the community who knew enough to intervene when an accident occurred.

Sadly, this is not the case in today's world. Very few have even the basic knowledge of how to treat an open wound or a snake bite, let along a broken bone or a heart attack. Hospitals are now overrun with "emergencies" that in the past would never have even required the attention of a doctor. A few years back four separate hospitals closed their doors in one year in Los Angeles due to excessive use of the emergency room trauma centers. Patients who truly needed the ER would not be able to get treatment due to the lack of care as the hospitals were overrun with non life threatening situations.

According to theguardian.com: "Up to 150,000 people a year could be dying unnecessarily because first aid is not widely enough known, a charity warns today. Situations where first aid could potentially make a difference include suffocations due to blocked airways, which claim 2,500 lives every year, and heart attacks, which kill 29,000.

St John Ambulance launched a new campaign to get more people to learn first aid skills. Its survey of more than 2,000 people found that 59% would not feel confident trying to save a life.

Meanwhile, almost a quarter (24%) would do nothing if they saw somebody struggling and would either wait for an ambulance to arrive or hope that a passerby knew first aid."

Curad, maker of adhesive bandages, in conjunction with the American Safety & Health Institute (ASHI), surveyed 200 first aid trainers concerning the general public's knowledge and preparedness when it comes to first aid. "When faced with a first aid emergency--no matter how minor or severe--our members say the biggest mistake people make is that they panic," indicates paramedic Ralph Shenefelt, general manager of ASHI. "By learning basic first aid and having the proper supplies to deal with minor first aid situations, the panic factor could be eased dramatically.

According to Wikipedia: "Skills of what is now known as first aid have been recorded throughout history, especially in relation to warfare, where the care of both traumatic and medical cases is required in particularly large numbers. The bandaging of battle wounds is shown on Classical Greek pottery from c. 500 BC, whilst the parable of the Good Samaritan includes references to binding or dressing wounds. There are numerous references to first aid performed within the Roman army, with a system of first aid supported by surgeons, field ambulances, and hospitals. Roman legions had the specific role of capsarii, who were responsible for first aid such as bandaging, and are the forerunners of the modern combat medic. Further examples occur through history, still mostly related to battle, with examples such as the Knights Hospitaller in the 11th century AD, providing care to pilgrims and knights in the Holy Land.

With technology comes more dependence on it's gifts and as can be seen from above, thousands are needlessly dying simply due to a lack of knowledge about basic first-aid skills. This is where this books come in. Not only will we be covering how to administer first-aid in a variety of situations, we will also be learning how this can be done in a more holistic, natural manner.

In this book we will learn about the natural treatment for such issues as burns, bleeding both minor and more severe, various types of poisonings, broken bone after care, snake bites, immediate life saving care for a heart attack or stroke victim, eye injuries, minor dental complaints and many more.

I will also be giving case histories where these tools have been used successfully, both on our clinic as well as from our patients who were taught these simple, historically proven techniques.

As always, please keep in mind that the care of a professional health care provider is sometimes required and we do not want you to make medical decisions on your own that may jeopardize yours or another life.

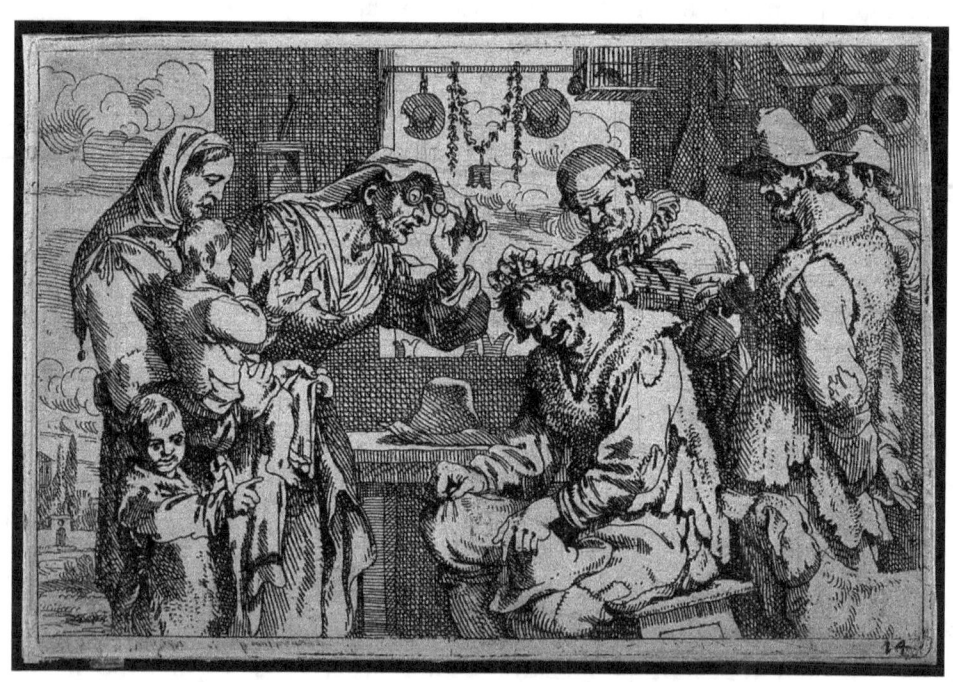

CHAPTER 2

BASIC FIRST-AID

2.1 Burns

This has to be one of the most common issues we have treated in the clinic as well as from family and friends. This can range for something as simple as a first degree sunburn to third degree house fires and electrical burns.

The American Burn Association states that:
- 44 percent of all admissions to burn centers result from fire or flame burns.
- 33 percent of all burn center admissions result from scalding injuries caused by wet or moist heat.
- Direct contact with a hot source accounts for nine percent of burn center admissions.
- Electrical burns account for four percent of burn center admissions.
- Chemical burns account for three percent of all burn center admissions.
- The remaining seven percent of burn center admissions are caused by other, miscellaneous sources.

The American Burn Association reports the following pediatric burn statistics for 2000:
- Scalding is the most common burn injury in children under four years old, accounting for 200,000 injuries per year.
- An estimated 50 percent of scalds are from spilled food and drinks, while the remainder are primarily from hot tap water and hot objects such as irons, stoves, and heaters.
- Each year, roughly 250,000 children under age 17 require medical attention for burn injuries.
- Roughly 15,000 children require hospitalization for burn injuries.

- About 1,100 children per year die from fires and burn injuries.

The American Burn Association states that of the 3,400 U.S. burn injury deaths each year:
- 2,550 of these deaths are a result of residential fires.
- 300 of these deaths result from vehicle crash fires.
- The remaining 550 result from other causes, such as flames, smoke inhalation, scalding, and electricity.

And finally ...

The Centers for Disease Control and Prevention provides the following statistics for costs related to burns:
- Males account for roughly $4.8 billion, or 64 percent, or total fire and burn-related costs each year, while females account for the remaining $2.7 billion, or 36 percent.
- Fatal burn and fire injuries cost roughly $3 billion, which accounts for two percent of the total cost of fatal injuries.
- Burn and fire hospitalization accounts for $1 billion, or one percent of hospitalized injury costs.
- Non-hospitalized burn and fire injuries account for two percent of non-hospitalized injury costs, or $3 billion.

As can be seen from the above statistics, so much of this could be avoided if we knew how to care for our own injuries. Of course, this does not negate the fact that there are times we would need the care of a qualified healthcare provider. This section is for those who do not have access to a hospital or another doctor.

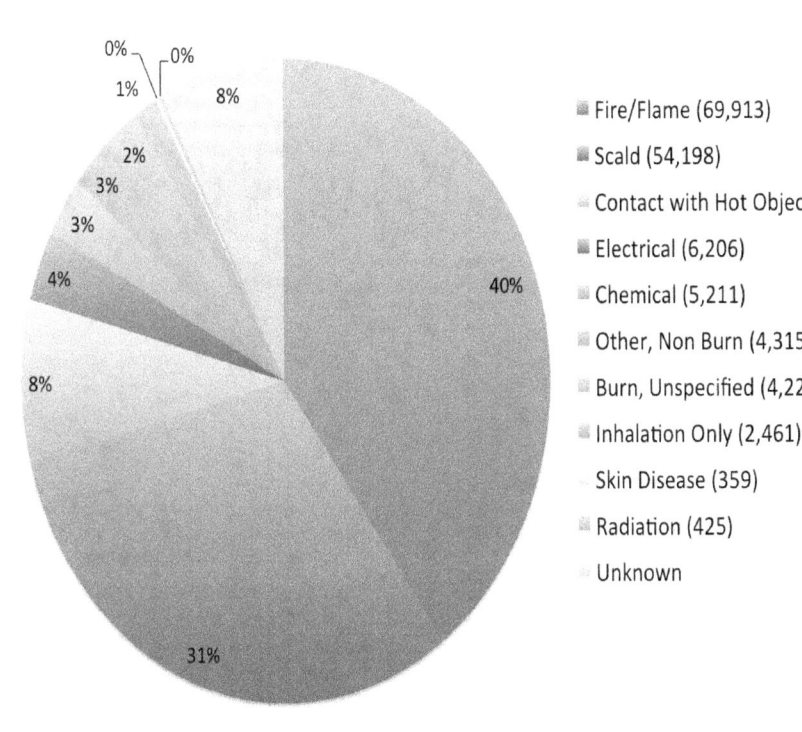

The good news is that there are wonderful history proven protocols that we can do to care for our injuries with natural holistic medicines. I will go over the varying degrees of burns, their types and the basic first aid for treating during an emergency.

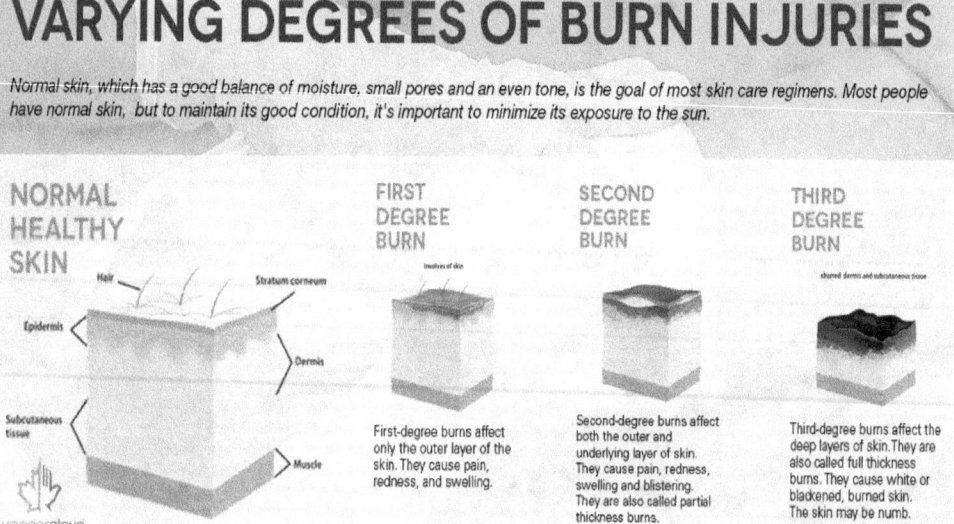

The above chart shows most burns are classified as first through third degree. There are higher classifications but that is beyond the scope of this book and they do REQUIRE a professionals assistance.

Types of first degree burns:

First-degree burns cause minimal skin damage. They are also called "superficial burns" because they affect the outermost layer of skin. Signs of a first-degree burn include:

- redness
- minor inflammation, or swelling
- pain
- dry, peeling skin occurs as the burn heals

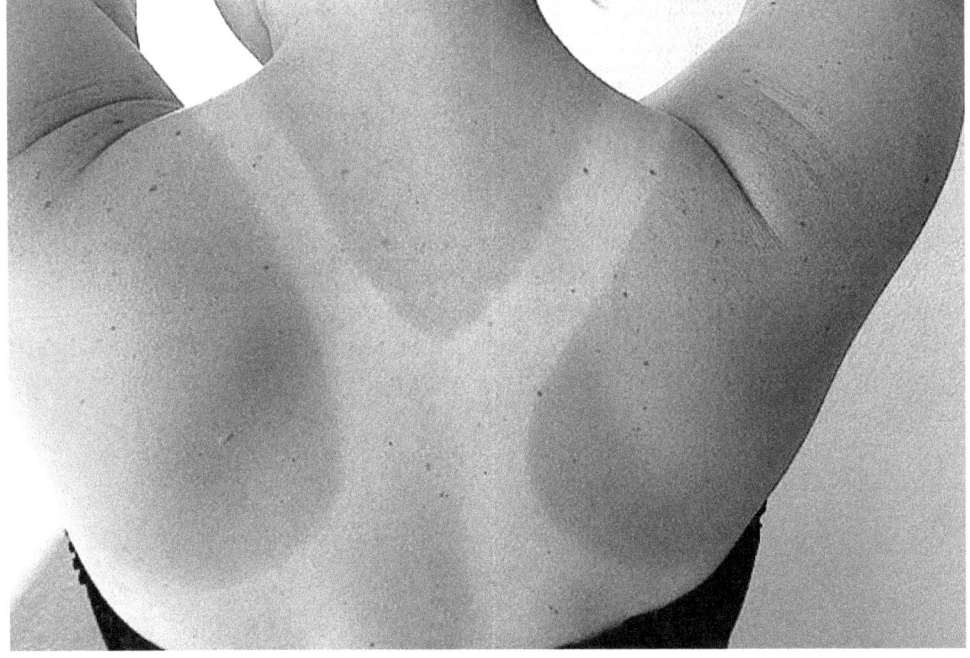

This burn affects only the top layer of skin, the signs and symptoms disappear once the skin cells shed. First-degree burns usually heal within 7 to 10 days without scarring.

CARE FOR FIRST DEGREE BURN:

The first thing you can do is to soak the burn in cool water. For pain and to aid in healing, the tried and true method used by most patients is a gel made from Aloe Vera. You can make this yourself from the fresh leaves of the plant or you can obtain the gels easily from most health food and pharmacy stores over the counter. Make sure NOT to use ice as this can make the damage worse. Do not use cotton balls as the fibers can stick to the burn possibly leading to infection.

Types of Second degree burns:

Second-degree burns are more serious because the damage extends beyond the top layer of skin. This type of burn causes the skin to blister and become extremely red and sore.

Some blisters pop open, giving the burn a wet or weeping appearance. Over time, thick, soft, scab-like tissue called fibrinous exudate may develop over the wound.

Due to the delicate nature of these wounds, keeping the area clean and bandaging it properly is required to prevent infection. This also helps the burn heal more quickly. As with first-degree burns, avoid cotton balls. Some second-degree burns take longer than three weeks to heal, but most heal within two to three weeks without scarring, but often with pigment changes to the skin.

Second Degree Burns

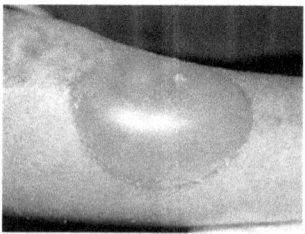

- Partial Thickness Burn
- Burns Epidermis and Dermis
- *Blisters forming is the key to DX*
- Mottled, Swelling, Wet, and Painful
- 3-4 Weeks to heal
- Cause Excessive Exposure to Sun, Radiation, Hot or Boiling Liquids, or Fire

CARE FOR SECOND DEGREE BURN:

To treat for this type of burn run it under cool water for 15 minutes or more. Aloe Vera will work with this type of burn but infection becomes a greater possibility so we opt for a preparation that is more effective at fighting a possible infection and does wonders for lowering the risk for scarring. This is a famous formula designed by Dr. Christopher and is called the burn ointment:

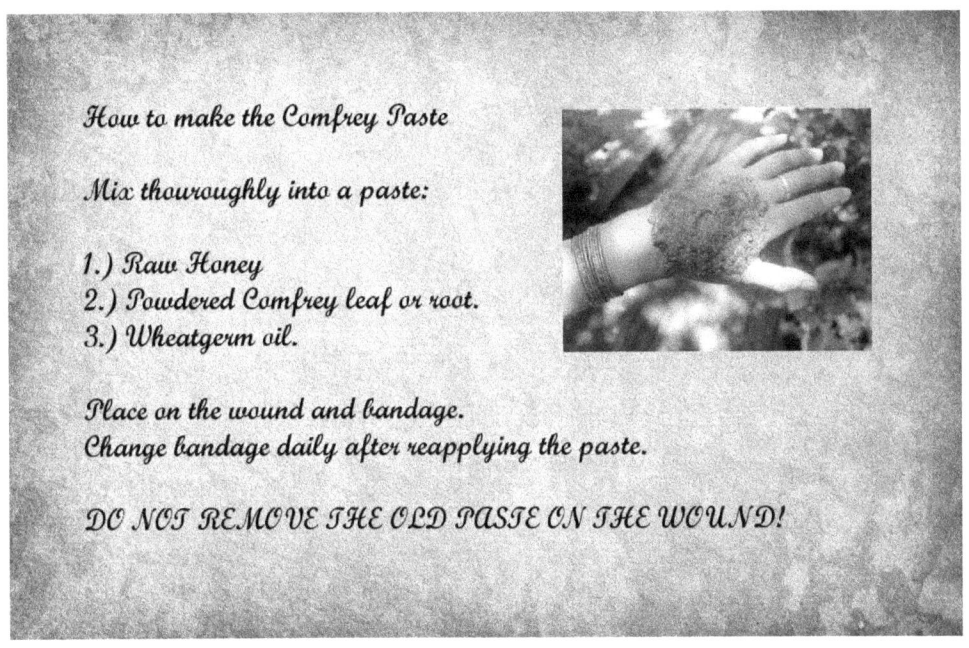

How to make the Comfrey Paste

Mix thouroughly into a paste:

1.) Raw Honey
2.) Powdered Comfrey leaf or root.
3.) Wheatgerm oil.

Place on the wound and bandage.
Change bandage daily after reapplying the paste.

DO NOT REMOVE THE OLD PASTE ON THE WOUND!

This is a very simple formula that has been used successfully for over 60 years. I have personally seen this remarkable mixture heal very serious burns with no scarring afterwards.

As you will notice, the main herb is Comfrey. As Dr. Christopher defined it, "Comfrey is one of the patriarchal herbs that I believe harkens back to the Garden of Eden. The Creator placed it on the Earth knowing that the human race was going to make a rough time of it and would need a universal salve for the wounds of war."

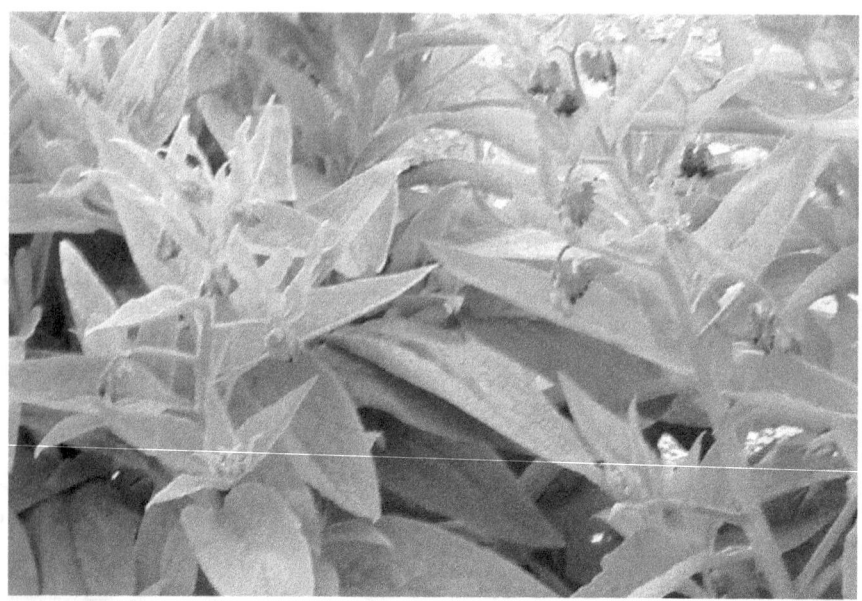

COMFREY

One of the most amazing properties of Comfrey is it's ability as a cell proliferate. This means that is able to cause cells to regrow very quickly. I have seen patient's broken arms heal in a third to half the time it commonly takes.

Some of the benefits of Comfrey include:

- Accelerate Wound Healing
- Relieves Back Pain
- Hydrates and repairs skin
- Boosts bone healthcare

For those who have read my book titled *Case Histories From A Successful Naturopathic Clinic,* you may remember the case of patient who had an advanced case of gangrene on his foot and was at a high risk for amputation. One of the main herbal formulas used contained a significant amount of Comfrey in it and the results were amazing. His foot, which had seriously decayed by the time he called (two months), completely regrew the flesh and muscle and left very little scar after months of treatment. Below are the before and after pictures. Please be aware the before is somewhat graphic.

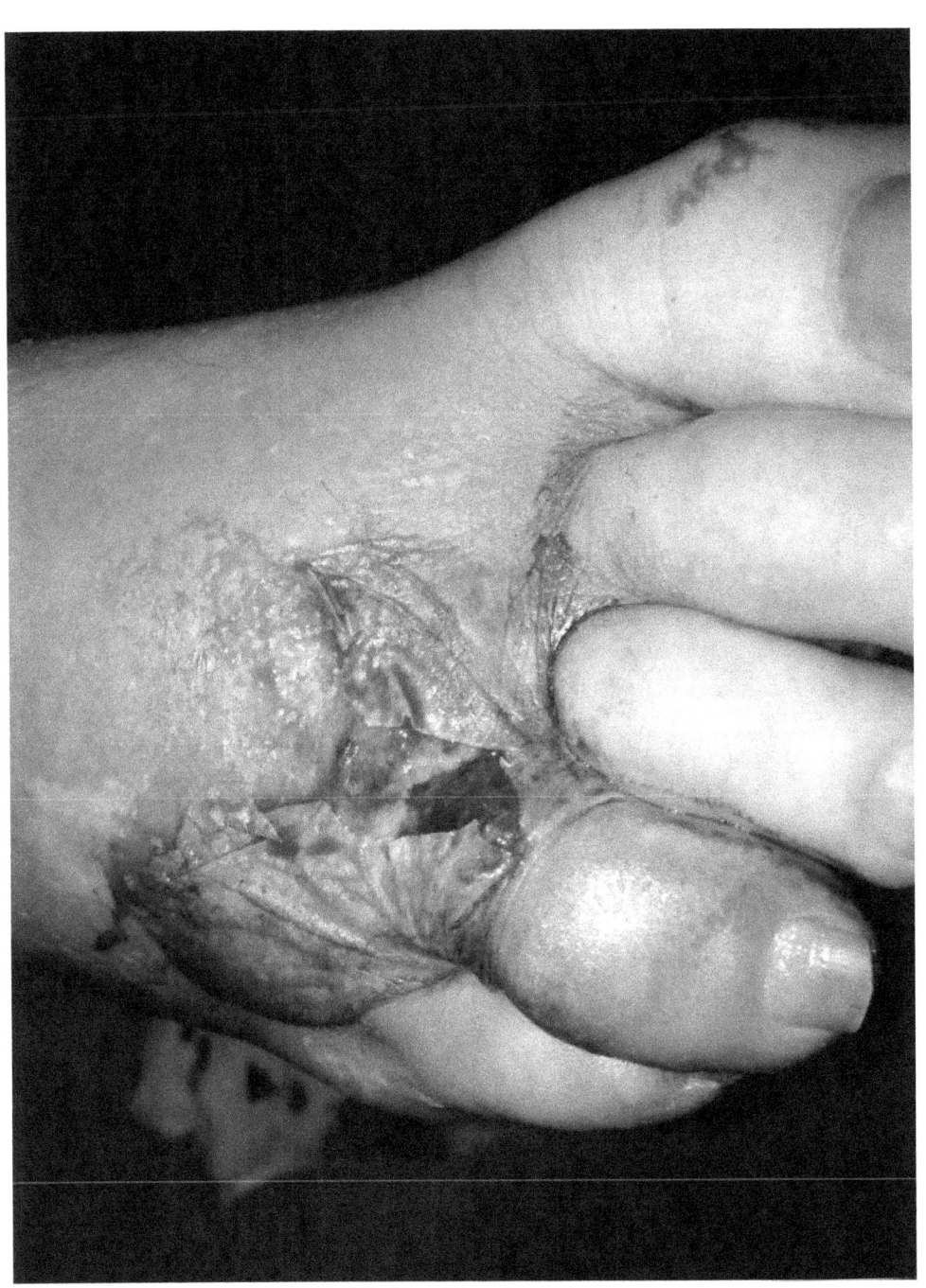

Before Treatment

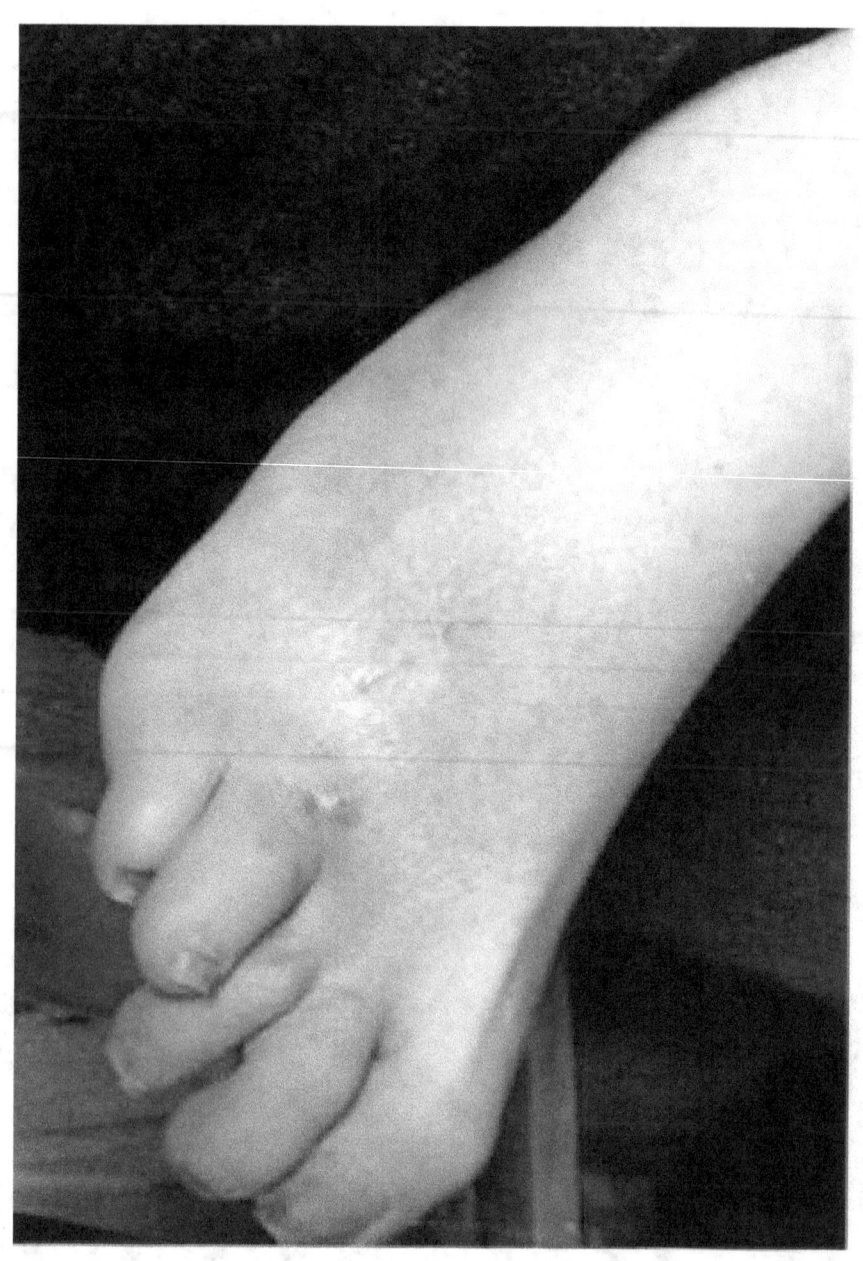

After several months of treatment

Types of Third degree burns:

Other than fourth degree burns, third degree burns are the most severe. This level of burn includes the most damage and may extend through every layer of skin. Risk of infection is usually very high. An interesting note is that these are often the least painful of burns as there can be extensive nerve damage.

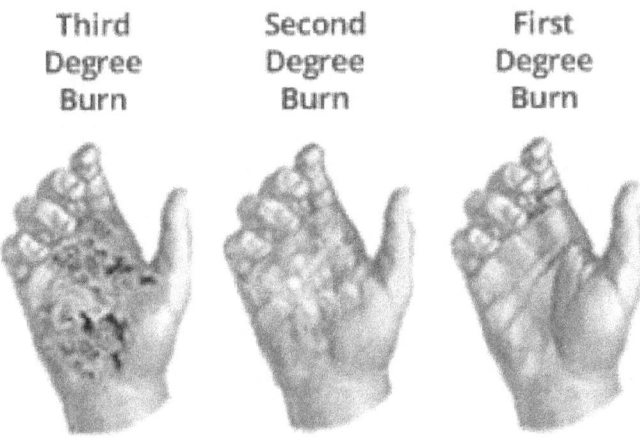

Depending on the cause, the symptoms third-degree burns can exhibit include:

- waxy and white color
- charring

- dark brown color
- raised and leathery texture
- blisters that do not develop

Without surgery, these wounds heal with severe scarring and contracture (where the limbs, fingers and such heal in a deformed manner and are not able to fully extend). While there is no set timeline for complete spontaneous healing for third-degree burns, we have seen healing occur more rapidly when holistic protocols are utilized.

As I discussed earlier, this can be a very serious burn and professional care is recommended. This book is for those who may not have easy access to a qualified healthcare provider. If you must treat it yourself then we find the Comfrey Paste formula or the B, F and C formula very effective. We would treat it by thickly coating the burn area with the paste or salve and wrapping it. It needs to be changed at least once a day as the body will absorb quite a bit of the salve. DO NOT remove the salve left over each time you change it. Simply reapply more salve on top of the old. You can also treat each day for possible infection by making sure the patient took either Dr. Christopher's Infection Formula at 4 capsules five times a day or by taking Garlic capsules at the same dosage. This may take weeks for the burn to heal, usually with little to no scarring.

2.2 Rashes

A rash is defined by Wikipedia as: A change of the human skin which affects its color, appearance, or texture. A rash may be localized in one part of the body, or affect all the skin. Rashes may cause the skin to change color, itch, become warm, bumpy, chapped, dry, cracked or blistered, swell, and may be painful.

The causes, and therefore treatments for rashes, vary widely. Diagnosis must take into account such things as the appearance of the rash, other symptoms, what the patient may have been exposed to, occupation, and occurrence in family members. The diagnosis may confirm any number of conditions. The presence of a rash may aid diagnosis; associated signs and symptoms are diagnostic of certain diseases. For example, the rash in measles is an erythematous, morbilliform, maculopapular rash that begins a few days after the fever starts. It classically starts at the head, and spreads downwards.

Skin rash facts
- *Rash* is not a specific diagnosis. Instead it refers to any sort of inflammation and/or discoloration that distorts the skin's normal appearance.
- Common rashes include eczema, poison ivy, hives, and athlete's foot.
- Infections that cause rashes may be fungal, bacterial, parasitic, or viral.
- Over-the-counter products may be helpful treatments for many skin rashes.
- Rashes lasting more than a few days that are unexplained should be evaluated by a doctor.

Some of the more common types of rashes:

Atopic dermatitis
- Seborrheic dermatitis
- Contact dermatitis
- Diaper rash
- Stasis dermatitis

- Psoriasis
- Hives
- Nummular eczema
- Drug eruptions
- Heat rash (miliaria)

Psoriasis is an autoimmune disorder and is therefore beyond the scope of this book. Please check out my book *Case Histories of a Successful Naturopathic Clinic* for more information.

Most of the rashes above fall within the realm of allergic reactions and yeast and fungus. I will cover in this section how to treat those conditions.

Allergy Type Rashes:

Let's start with **allergic** types of rashes. These are very common and are often very simple to treat. As a Naturopath it is my inclination to treat the root cause (meaning why are you allergic to something in the first place) but the scope of this book is mainly for first aid treatments.

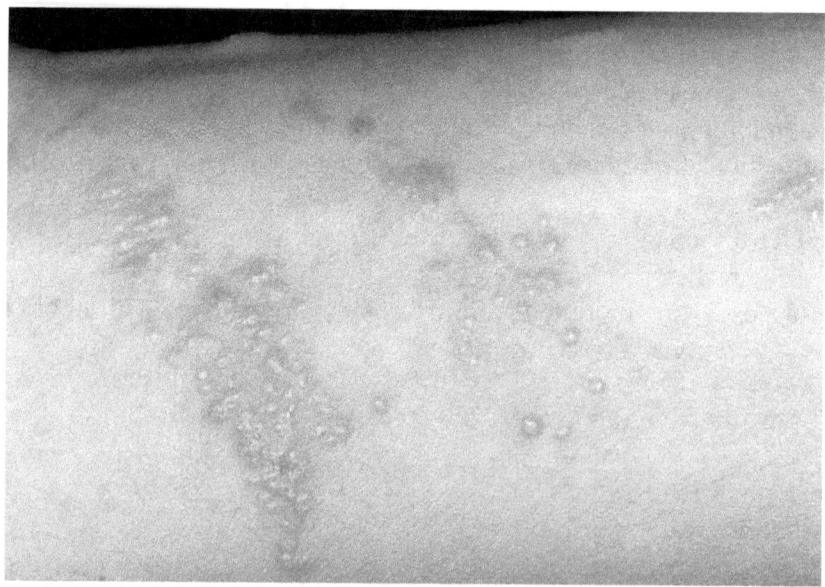

Poison Oak

One of the most common types of allergic rashes are contact dermatitis. Contact dermatitis is a rash that is brought on either by contact with a specific chemical to which the patient is uniquely allergic or with a substance that directly irritates the skin. Some chemicals are both irritants and allergens. This rash tends to be weepy and oozy and affects the parts of the skin which have come in direct contact with the offending substance. Common examples of allergic contact dermatitis are poison ivy, poison sumac, poison oak (same chemical, different plant) and reactions to costume jewelry containing nickel.

We use two different herbal aids to treat both the itch and the rash itself. The first is something we call Green Salve. It is made from a combination of Comfrey, Chickweed and Plantain. Many years ago this was a school project of mine and it was found to be so effective we continue to use it to this day in the clinic. It is made with equal parts of each of the herbs in an olive oil and bees wax base.

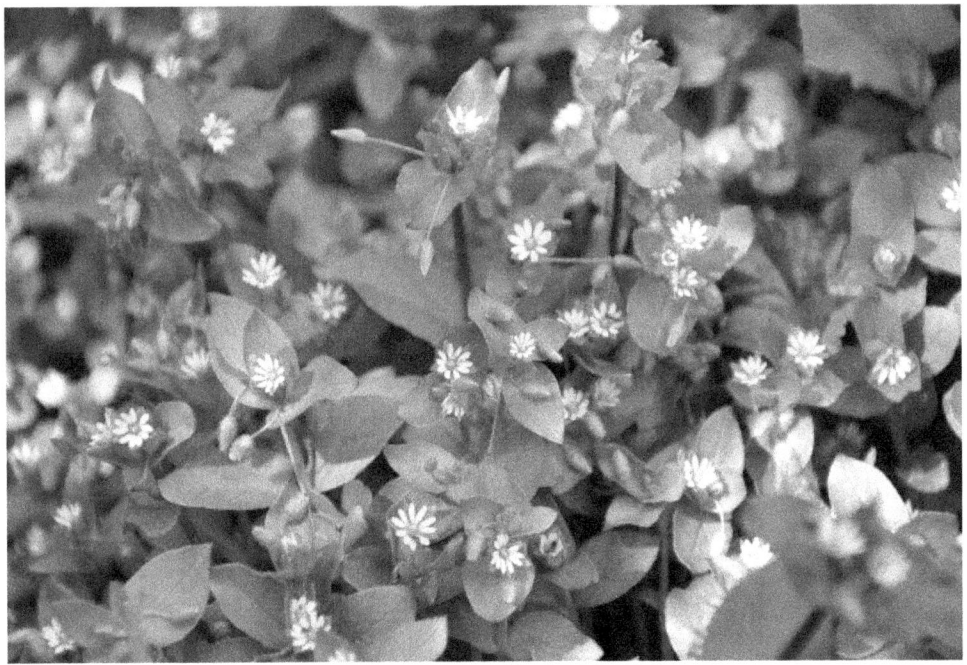

Chickweed (Stellaria Media)

We discussed earlier that Comfrey is a wonderful cell proliferate, meaning it has the ability to cause cells to regrow quickly. Chickweed has a wonderful reputation for soothing skin irritations.

Some of the benefits of Chickweed include:

- Prevents inflammation
- Encourages weight loss
- Alleviates respiratory problems
- Speeds up healing

Plantain:

There are two types of Plantain and both have similar properties and can be used interchangeably:

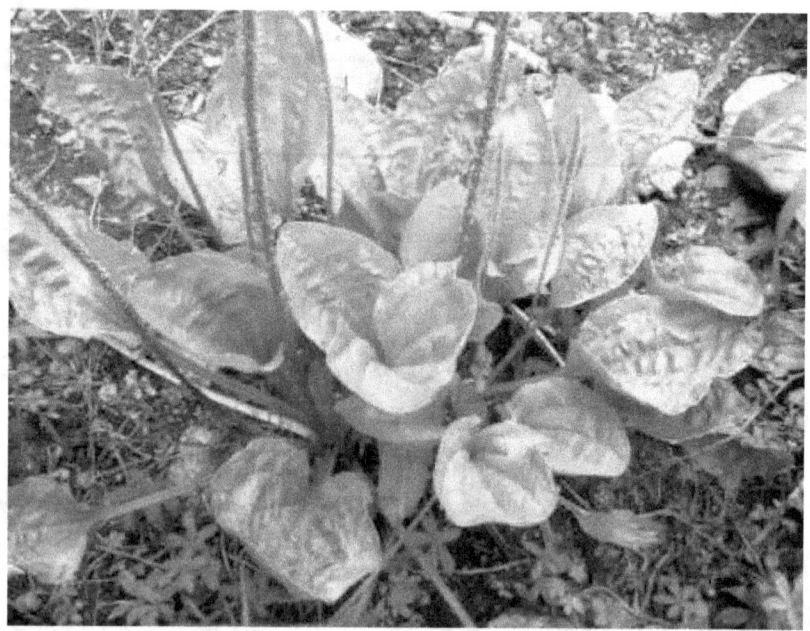

Plantago Major

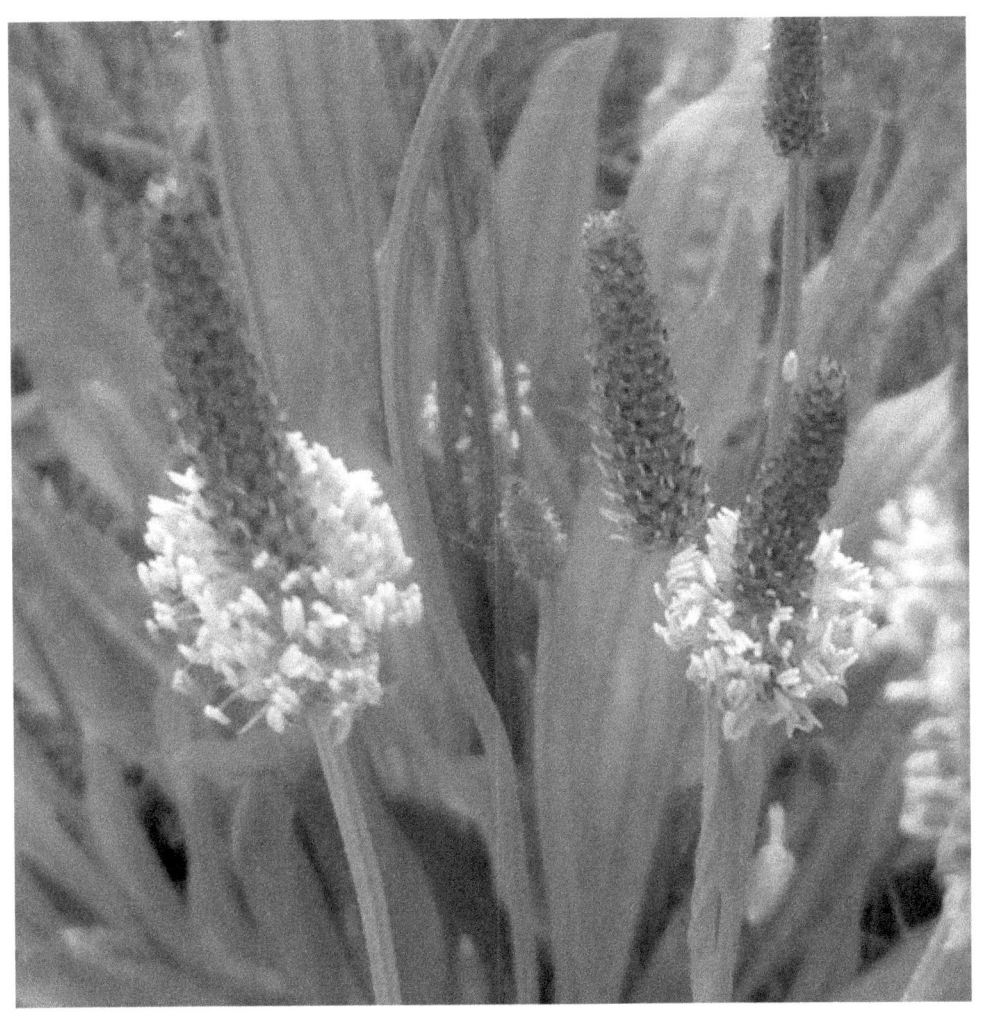

Plantago Lanceolata

Plantain Benefits:

- Respiratory infections.
- Heals cuts
- Treats constipation.
- Relieves boils and acne
- Treats insect bites and stings.
- Soothes irritated eyes.

- Treats burns.
- Relief for coughs and colds..
- Helps eczema and psoriasis.
- Good for the digestion.
- Soothes hemorrhoids.
- Treats mouth ulcers.

All of the above herbs can also be used as an oil or as a poultice. To prepare the Green Salve as a salve take the three equal parts (by weight) of the herbs mentioned and cover them in a pan completely with the olive oil. Simmer on low heat for about 20 to 25 minutes. Then strain out the herbs (after you let it cool for a bit) and keep the oil.

Now place the oil back in the pan and put it back on low heat. Start to add beeswax a little at a time and periodically test the oil in a spoon to see if it turns to a soft salve. You do this by letting the oil in the spoon cool for a minute. If it turns into a soft waxy salve then you should be fine. Please be aware that if you add too much wax then when the salve cools it will become a very hard block and difficult to use. Apply it as often as needed throughout the day for itch relief.

This is **NOT** to be used for fungal type rashes. I will discuss that issue later in this section.

HERBADYNE:

Another formula we have used with great success is a tincture (alcohol based) we call Herbadyne. It's original name was Jethro Kloss herbal liniment. It is considered the herbal sister to Betadine or Iodine. It has been very effective against such issues as poison oak, ivy, sumac as well as against the shingles virus and it's lesions. It is made with Myrrh, Golden seal and cayenne pepper. The beauty of a tincture is it's ability to last long term. I know of someone who likes to collect medieval tinctures. They were created around year 1450. They are still as good to this day as they were made with an alcohol base.

To make this formula;

Ingredients are 2 ounces of powdered Myrrh, one ounce powdered Golden seal, ½ ounce of powdered cayenne and one quart of 100 proof vodka.

Combine all of the herbs and alcohol in a glass jar, cap tightly and keep it in a cool, shaded area for 14 days. Shake at least once each day. Strain it and keep the alcohol in a dark bottle and store in a cool place.

As stated, we have used it very successful for most scrapes and rashes. It can help with fungal rashes as well. We have seen it begin to clear up poison oak as well as shingles within 12 hours. Just apply frequently throughout the day. We use it for all types of scrapes and cuts, to both treat and to prevent infection.

Fungal Type Rashes:

Fungal type rashes include yeast (also seen in diaper rashes) impetigo, and ringworm. Fungal infections are fairly common. Yeasts are botanically related to fungi and can cause skin rashes. These tend to affect folds of skin (like the skin under the breasts or the groin). They look fiery red and have pustules (blisters) around the edges.

Fungal rashes are not commonly acquired from dogs or other animals. They seem to be most easily acquired in gyms, showers, pools, or locker rooms, or from other family members. If a fungus has been repeatedly treated without success, it is worthwhile considering the possibility that it was never really a fungus to start with but rather a form of eczema.

Ringworm, fungal

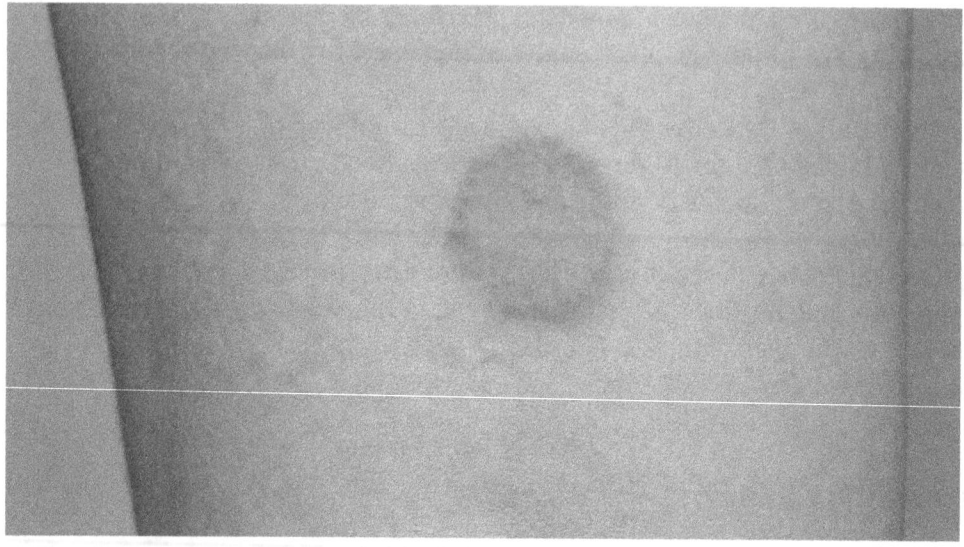

These types of rashes include:

- Most cases of diaper rash
- Ringworm
- Candida rashes
- Tinea
- Athletes foot
- Jock itch

A major cause of these rashes is a weakened immune system.

Treatment here is different since fungal rashes are basically a form of "plant" and we do not want to give it any moisture. There are many wonderful alternative treatments and each rash may require a different protocol.

Treatment #1:

One of the best treatment we have found for stubborn fungal rashes is the use of a solution made from distilled water and Braggs Apple Cider Vinegar.

We usually start off with a 50/50 solution of distilled water and Braggs. Scrub the rash several times a day. It can show a difference within one day. **DO NOT STOP** until the rash is completely gone. If needed, you can do a stronger solution of the Apple cider vinegar but that depends on how sensitive your skin is and how well it tolerates the vinegar.

Treatment #2:

One herb that has been very successful with diaper rash, as well as other fungal types is Black Walnut. We use it in an olive oil and beeswax salve.

Black walnut benefits:

- Supports healthy skin in cases of pimples, skin blemishes, acne breakouts, Psoriasis and eczema.
- It can banish warts.
- Kills parasites.
- Kills fungal infections.
- Improve digestion
- Even found to fight cancer!
- Support heart health.
- Soothes a sore throat.

Not bad, eh? More effective than any pharmaceutical I am aware of. Apply everyday and put a bandage over and change each day. In the case of diaper rash, simply apply several times a day without a bandage. Please be aware that many children and some adults are **VERY** sensitive to the latex and glue in bandages and I have seen cases where the damage from the bandage was worse than the original issue.

2.3 Bites and Stings

With warmer weather comes our neighbors from the forests and fields. Insects and other creatures such as snakes come out to do what comes natural to them but often a torment to the humans. Here we are going to go over some of the things you can do at home to remedy these occurrences.

There are multitudes of different little ones out there who can leave their mark. There are bees, wasps, bed bugs, ticks, mosquitoes, spiders, snakes, etc. Let's look at the symptoms and what we can do for them.

- Bedbugs leave a small bite mark on the skin that is red and itchy or causes a serious allergic reaction.
- Bee stings cause a red skin bump with white around it.
- Flea bites leave an itchy welt on the skin, often on the ankles and legs.
- Mosquitoes leave a raised, itchy pink skin bump or in rare cases a severe allergic reaction.
- Spider bites cause minor symptoms like red skin, swelling, and pain at the site or very serious symptoms that need emergency care.
- Ticks can carry Lyme disease and their bite can leave (only 20% of the time) a rash that looks like an expanding bull's-eye.

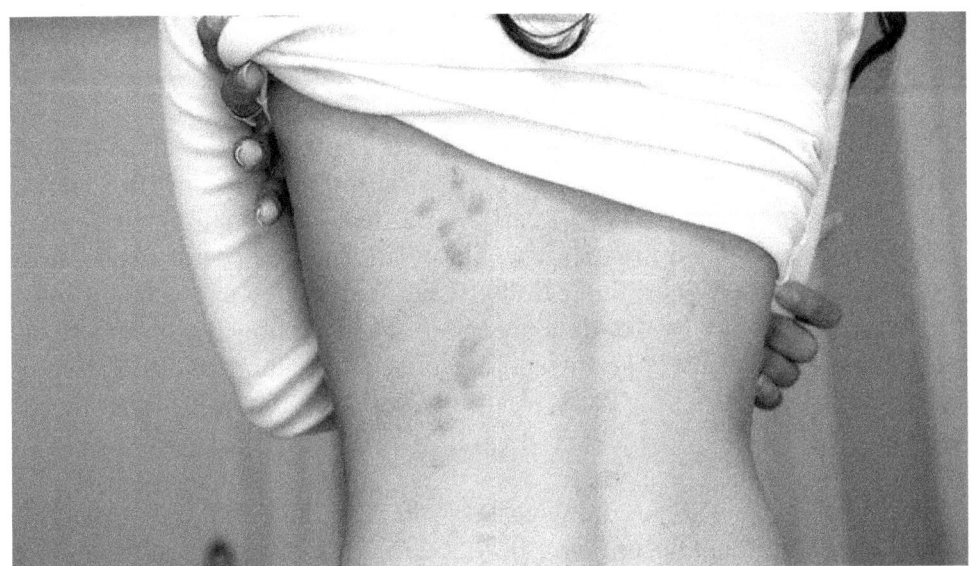
Bed bug bite marks

Usually, the reason bed bug bites become an issue is due to you having an allergic reaction to them. Not everyone has this issue. But if you do, it can be very simple to treat.

First thing of course is to manage the itch. Scratching can lead to greater damage and infection. Here are some simple, at home herbal treatments:

Poke: The skin is an indicator of toxicity in the body. Poke is a good aid for skin problems. It is also good for "the itch" in cases of scabies. Anytime you have skin which doesn't eliminate properly along with vitiated blood, you can well use Poke. It is said to be a great eliminator of toxins out of the system. Usually the glands are not performing properly in these conditions so the herb works on both areas. It is often used in chronic eczema, syphilitic eruptions, psoriasis, varicose veins and leg ulcers.

A mixture of chickweed, olive oil and bees wax makes a great anti-ointment.

Our **Herbadyne** tincture described above works well as it also kills the scabies and bed bugs and relives the itching from them. A solution of distilled water and Braggs Apple Cider Vinegar, 50/50 solution, bathed over the bite can also help relive the itch.

So what do you do if it does becomes infected? The **Green Salve** mentioned earlier works very well for drawing out the poison and the infection. Back many years ago, when I was still early in my lessons on natural first aid, I was bitten by a spider. I thought it would be a great idea to put fresh garlic on the wound. Not a good thing to do. Fresh garlic juice can actually burn the skin. The next day I woke up to a very serious infection and open sore on my hand. Garlic is a wonderful anti-bacterial and natural antibiotic when taken internally or used topically in an olive oil base, but NOT directly on the skin.

I immediately went out and did what I should have done in the first place. I looked for some Plantain growing in the yard. This plant, as shown in the previous section grows all around the world and throughout the United States. Most consider it a weed and that is a shame and a loss. It is wonderful at wound care as it is very efficient at drawing out the infection and sealing the wound quickly.

I made a poultice of the fresh plant that I had gathered. To do this I placed the fresh plants, after I had crushed them and broken up the leaves, into a pan of water. I steeped them at a low temperature for about twenty minutes or so. I then took them out, and after a little cooling so they would not scald, I placed them soaking directly onto the wound. I then wrapped it with a cloth bandage to keep the wet plant material on the wound. I left it on overnight. There are occasions where you will need to change it a couple of times a day.

When I woke the next morning I removed the bandage. I was shocked at the change. Not only was the redness of the infection gone but so was the pus itself. The wound had also closed and was well on it's way to being healed.

SPIDER BITES

Since we're on the subject of spiders, let's talk about treating these dreaded and often scary injuries. There are definitely occasions when you need to seek proper medical care such as in the case of the brown recluse or the black widow and I am not advocating doing this on your own. But ... there are also occasions when you may not have access to a qualified healthcare provider and you need to take the situation into your own hands.

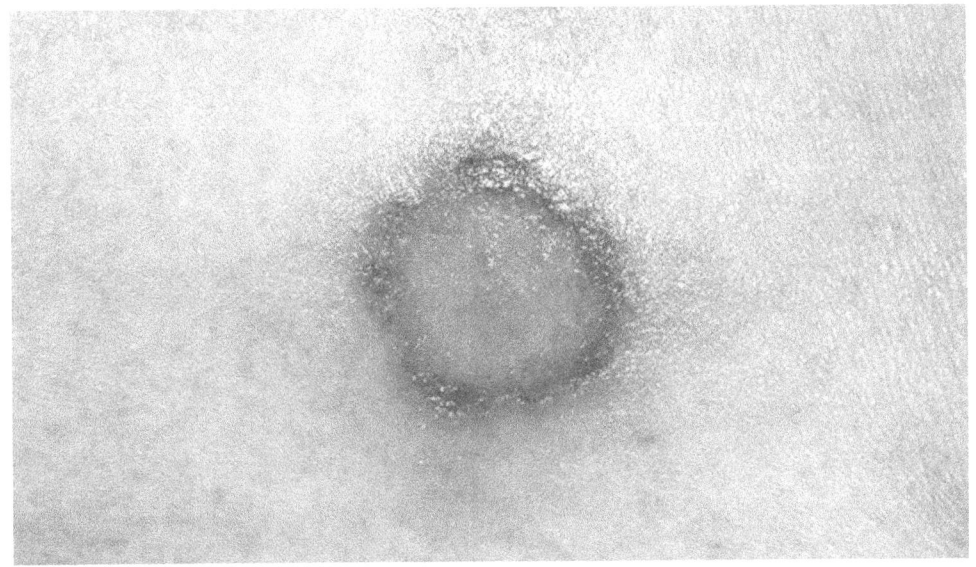

Example of a spider bite

One of the first things you can do is use the above poultice with Plantain. It is amazing at drawing out the poison. I also highly recommend using Poke root in the poultice and orally. You can put a dropper full or more of the Poke root onto the wound before you put the Plantain plant material on top of it. Poke, while it can cause you to throw up, if taken carefully, will not cause it and will help to neutralize the poison internally. At the time of the bite you can take a dropper full every half hour to an hour for at least five hours orally.

As stated earlier, you may need to change the poultice several times during the day to be most effective for drawing out the poison. After about a day you can start using salve like the green salve mentioned earlier. But again, seek medical aid if needed.

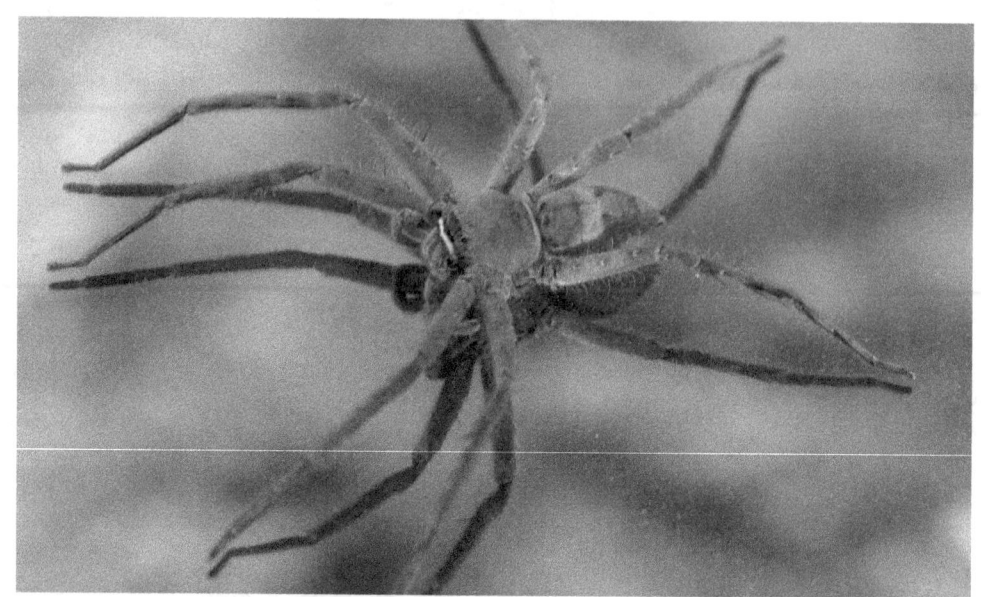

Brown Recluse spider

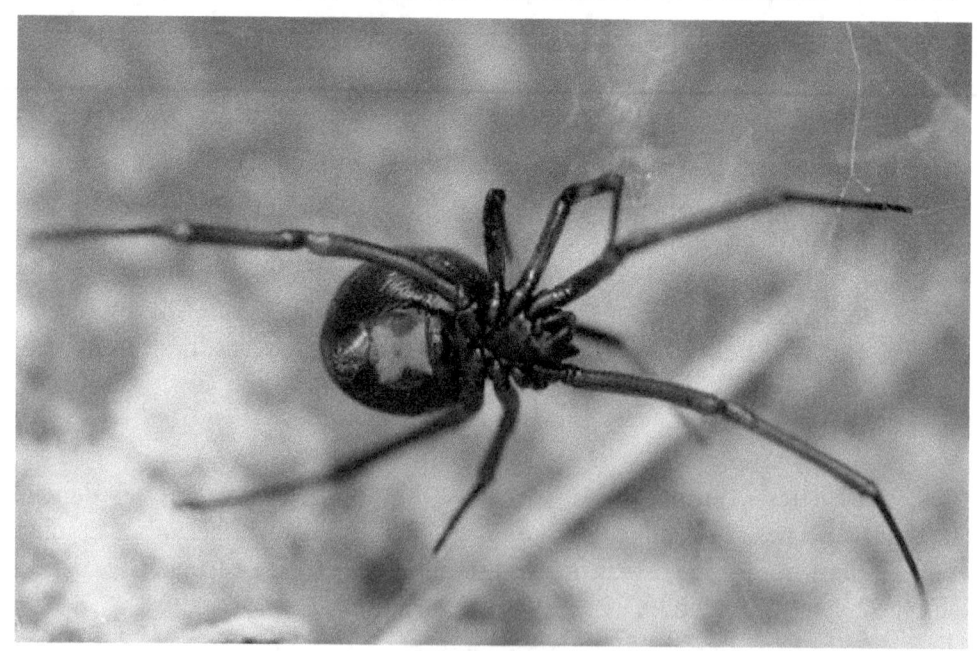

Black Widow spider

A good start is to also avoid being bitten or stung. There are a variety of natural insect repellents. As we go on our outings and picnics this summer, we dread the thought of insects: their stings, bites, annoyances, and the like. We invest in gallons of insect repellents which are expensive and possibly toxic. It is our purpose here to suggest some natural remedies to the problem of being bugged. Some of the simplest insect repellents can be made from our local herbs.

Chamomile and **Yarrow** are two of the best insect repellents in the field. Make a tea of either of these and wash the skin with them and insects will avoid you like the plague. This includes flies, mosquitoes, and their ilk. Because the cosmetic industry uses chaparral as an antiseptic lotion for insect bites, the tea of chaparral may also be tried as a repellent. A member of the family that includes potatoes, cayenne, and eggplant, also includes tobacco, which was used as a successful insect repellent for centuries. In fact, the Indians gave White man tobacco in order to drive them away from the continent. That is why we are taken aback at the reference to Indians smoking a "peace pipe" containing tobacco.

Feverfew: A tincture of the herb, applied locally, is used to relieve pain and swelling caused by bites of insects and vermin. An effective insect repellant is claimed by adding two teaspoonfuls of tincture to one half pint of cold water and then sponging any exposed parts of the body with it.

Chiggers: These are the scourge of the midwest. To repel them, use the aforementioned herbs. To allay the itch produced by their bites, either Chickweed or plantain ointment can be applied. Plantain is an excellent remedy to apply to the site of the bite. It is a blood purifier that will even rally to the occasion of a scorpion bite. It will reduce the red streaks of blood poisoning like no man-made remedy can.

Crushed Onions: Ant bites stop stinging with a poultice of crushed onions.

Pennyroyal: The oil of pennyroyal is a first-rate protection against insect bites (mosquitoes, gnats, and other similar winged pests). It should not be used during pregnancy.

SNAKE BITES:

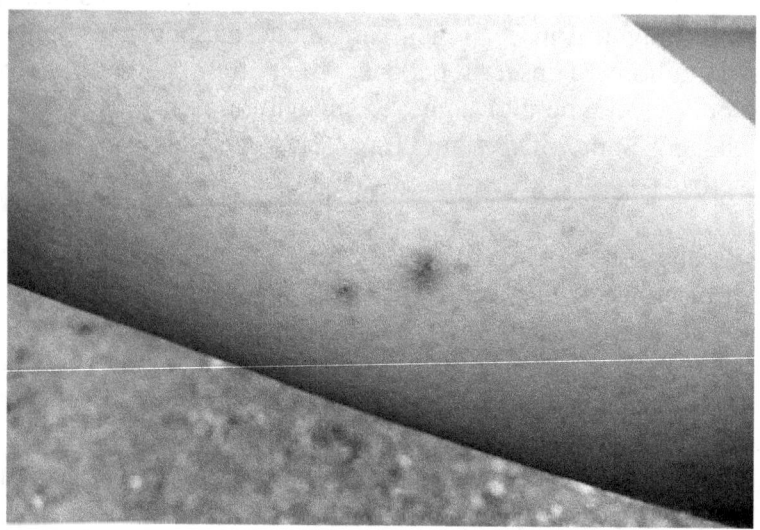

Snake bite

Needless to say, this can often be another occasion when you may want to opt for a qualified healthcare professional. But, as stated, before, that may not be an option. So what are some of the statistics on being bitten by a snake?

As stated by Wikipedia: The United States has about 20 species of venomous snakes, which include 16 species of rattlesnakes, two species of coral snakes, one species of cottonmouth (or water moccasin), and one species of copperhead. At least one species of venomous snake is found in every state except Hawaii and Alaska.

It has been estimated that 7,000–8,000 people per year receive venomous snake bites in the United States, and about five of those people die. Most fatal bites are attributed to the eastern diamondback rattlesnake and the western diamondback rattlesnake. The copperhead accounts for more cases of venomous snake bite than any other North American species; however, its venom is the least toxic, so its bite is seldom fatal.

Venomous snakes are distributed unevenly throughout the United States — the vast majority of snake bites occur in warm weather states. States like

Florida and Texas have a wide variety and large population of venomous snakes. Bites from venomous snakes are extremely rare in the states near the Canada–US border. Maine, for example, has only one species (timber rattlesnake); it is rarely seen, and then only in the southern part of the state, but the species is likely extirpated in Maine, with the last sighting in 1901

The good news is that only about 10% of snake bites are fatal. For example, if a rattle snake does bite you, there is only a 15% you even received any venom from the bite and only a 1% chance you will die from it without receiving any care. The very young, elderly and those with a weakened immune system are the most at risk.

HERBAL AIDES:

So, what can be done if you are bitten? Here again, we go back to our champion of the bites and stings ... Plantain.

Plantain: The American Indians used Plantain for a variety of ills. It is said that a South Carolina Indian was given a reward for the information that Plantain was the chief remedy for the cure of rattlesnake bite. Indians are said to have applied a poultice of Plantain for battle bruises and for drawing out snake poisons. The Shoshone Indians made poultices of the whole plant and applied them to the bruises of battles. In some cases, the poultices are combined with the foliage of wild clematis. The Indians of southern Massachusetts applied the leaves both for wounds and for snakebites. The Chippewas used it for inflammation, and as an application to draw out a splinter.

Testimonials:

1. Plantain Leaves and a Sting on the Neck: A 2-year-old was stung on the neck, and the part swelled to enormous size. Again, the remedy was simple, yet wonderfully effective: four plantain leaves were bruised and bound around the neck, and within one hour there was no sign that anything had been wrong with the child.

2. Plantain to the Rescue Again: We have gone on a house call where the hand and arm were swollen up and up the enlarged arm was a red streak with a lump under the arm pit. The individual had blacked out with pain from

the wasp sting and swelling. It was early spring and the plantain was not up, so I could not use it fresh. I put plantain ointment, about the size of a dollar, over the sting and within a half an hour the pain was gone. This was in the morning, and they reported back later that the swelling and red streak were gone by afternoon and this boy was out playing ball later that day.

OTHER HERBAL AIDES:

Echinacea: The Omaha Poncas used Echinacea as a basic herb for a variety of ailments. The fresh root was placed on toothaches until the pain subsided. It was used on enlarged glands--like mumps. A smoke fumigant of Echinacea was used to treat headaches, snakebite.

Black Cohosh: The bruised root, applied to the wound, was used by the Indians as an antidote for snakebite, with the juice in small amounts taken internally, apparently by chewing bits of the root.

2.4 Lice

Louse - a general name for various degraded parasitic insects; the true lice that infest mammals belong to the suborder Anoplura Capitus, or head louse; P. Corporis, the body or clothes louse; and Phthirus, or crab louse which lives in the hair upon the pubis, and the eye lashes and eye brows.

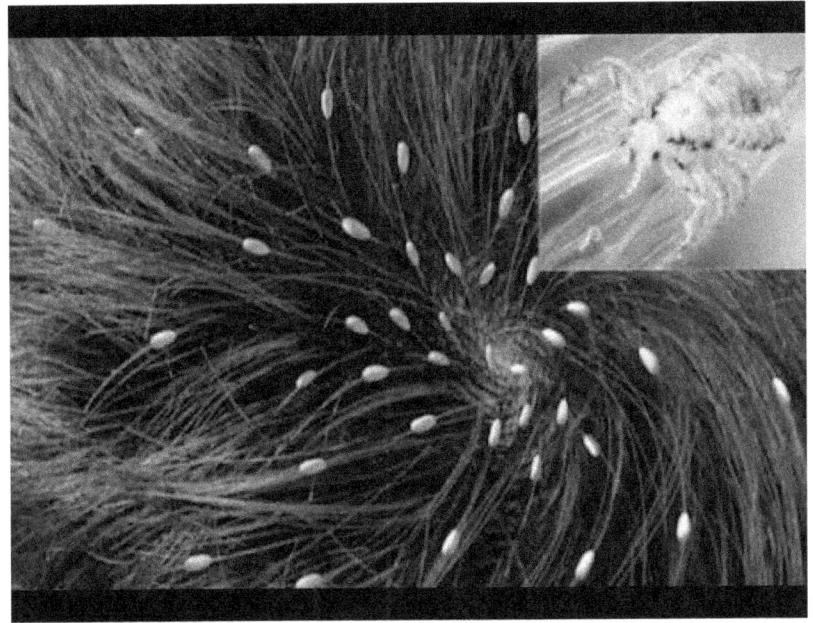

Lice

The causal organisms of typhus fever, relapsing fever, trench fever, and possibly plague are transmitted by the bites of lice. Head lice will never stay around the body that is completely healthy, with no toxins or accumulations of mucus. Lice and all body vermin are scavengers and cannot exist long with clean healthy cells. Keep the bowels clean, stay on a mucusless diet, bathe daily, and lice will not appear.

As recommended by Dr. Christopher: For quick relief (working on the effect) is to bathe the head or body parts covered with lice with straight apple cider vinegar, oil of garlic or walnut (leaf, bark or nut husk) tea. When lice are detected in the family, see that in addition to working on the cause (cleaning the bowel and blood stream) and staying on a mucusless diet, work on the effect itself as suggested here. See that fresh clothes--inner and outer clothing--are changed daily. All of these clothes should be washed with a good biodegradable soap with a cup or more of apple cider vinegar to each washerful of clothes. Change the bed linen each day. Spray the room with tea made of six parts chaparral, three parts black walnut leaf or bark, one part lobelia and to each pint of the spray add some lavender oil or oil of mint to give fragrance.

Another general recommendation by Dr. Christopher included a specific treatment when they are present. Create an infusion of six parts hyssop (Hyssopus officinalis), one part walnut leaves or inner bark (Juglans cinerea), one half part cinnamon bark powder, one half part cloves powder, one half part lobelia, and one half part ginger (Zingiber officinale).

DOSAGE: 1/2 cup (more or less according to age) three times in a day, taken orally. Make fomentation over the head with the same formula, and in other areas infected; covering the fomentation with a plastic or rubber cap at night. Do this six days a week as many weeks as needed to clear up the condition.

Please also remember, a clean house and clean body are not to the liking of our scavenger friends, lice, mites, fleas, etc.

2.5 Warts

As defined by Wikipedia: **Warts** are typically small, rough, hard growths that are similar in color to the rest of the skin. They typically do not result in other symptoms, except when on the bottom of the feet, where they may be painful. While they usually occur on the hands and feet, they can also affect other locations. One or many warts may appear. They are not cancerous.

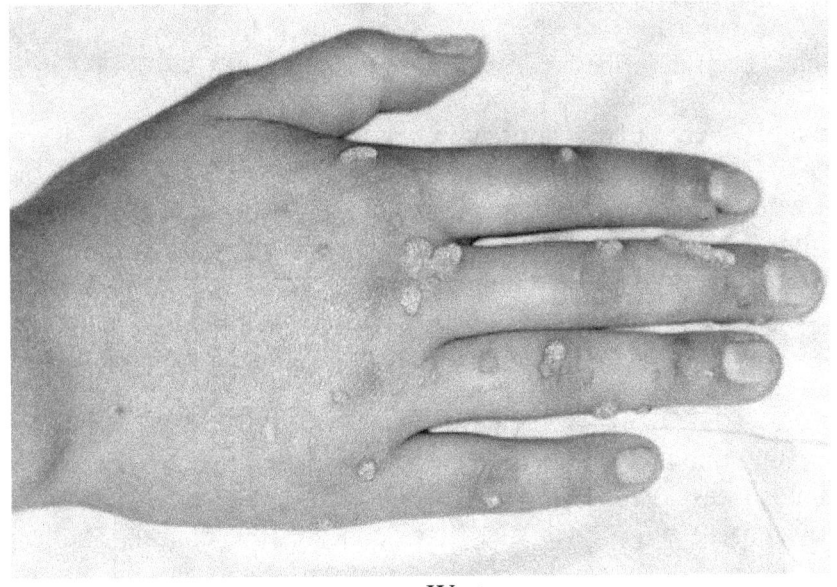
Warts

Warts are caused by infection with a type of human papillomavirus (HPV). Factors that increase the risk include use of public showers, working with meat, eczema and a weak immune system. The virus is believed to enter the body through skin that has been damaged slightly. A number of types exist, including "common warts", plantar warts, "filiform warts", and genital warts. Genital warts are often sexually transmitted

As with most human conditions, warts are usually the result of a nutritional deficiency (most often potassium) and they should be treated internally, as well as externally.

Without treatment, most types of warts resolve in months to years. A number of treatments may speed resolution including salicylic acid applied to the skin and cryotherapy. In those who are otherwise healthy, they do not typically result in significant problems. Treatment of genital warts differs from that of other types.

Warts are very common, with most people being infected at some point in their lives. The estimated current rate of non-genital warts among the general population is 1–13%. They are more common among young people. The estimated rate of genital warts in sexually active women is 12%. Warts have been described at least as far back as 400 BC by Hippocrates

Fortunately, there are a large number of natural cures for warts. As recommended by Dr. Christopher: "The warts, moles and skin blemishes are helped externally and are often cleared up by using the white milk from dandelions and/or from milkweed. Applying castor oil or garlic oil to the area several times a day and taping a piece of gauze soaked with this oil over the wart during the night will aid in clearing the condition. The use of a clove of garlic cut in half (or mashed or grated) and kept over the wart all night until it is gone has aided many."

Black walnut tincture and the following combination tincture have been used with such success that a number of people swear by them. The combination tinctures consists of Blue vervain, Black cohosh, Blue cohosh, Skullcap and Lobelia herbs [Ear and Nerve Tincture] in equal parts, using 90 proof or stronger alcohol as a base.

Potassium Deficiency for Warts and Moles: When cysts or tumors grow in places where they can be seen outside the body, often we react by having them cut out. This defeats healing by working on the effect instead of the cause. You can cut cysts out, tumors off, and burn warts off (which are also a potassium deficiency), or get rid of as many moles as you wish, but unless you go to the cause, they will grow back again, and you may end up with as many or more cysts, tumors, moles as before. Different signs of potassium deficiency will keep popping out on the body because the condition that needs correcting is on the inside. You have to go into the cause, Dr. Christopher always insisted, which is the way we have been eating.

Potassium sources: There are several ways to receive your potassium. Dr. Bernard Jensen sells a potassium broth made from dehydrated vegetables. Dr. Bronner makes a similar, excellent product. You can also make your own potassium broth by simmering equal parts of red potatoes, celery, carrots, onions, and herbs to taste. Raw vegetable and fruit juices also flood the system with potassium.

2.6 Abrasions/bruises

As defined by Wikipedia: An **abrasion** is a partial thickness wound caused by damage to the skin and can be superficial involving only the epidermis to deep, involving the deep dermis. Abrasions usually involve minimal bleeding. Mild abrasions, also known as *grazes* or *scrapes*, do not scar or bleed because the dermis is left intact, but deep abrasions that disrupt the normal dermal structures may lead to the formation of scar tissue. A more traumatic abrasion that removes all layers of skin is called an avulsion.

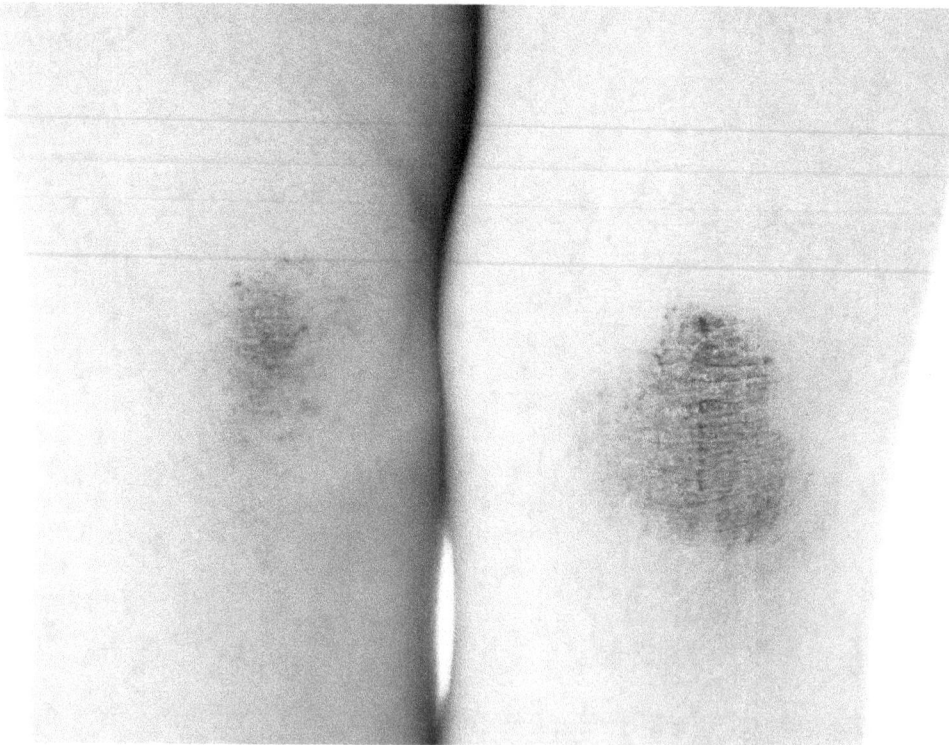

An abrasion

Like much that we have discussed in this chapter, these are usually very simple to treat naturally with little risk of infection.

The first thing I teach my students is to make sure and treat the open scrape with a herbal disinfectant such as Herbadyne. I gave you the instructions on how to make it on page 26. Apply at least once a day, the more the better. It will sting just like Iodine but I have never in over 20 years seen anyone become infected after it's proper use. Once the Herbadyne is applied I then put a healing salve on top of it.

As mentioned before, one of the best aids for scrapes and such is the paste made from Comfrey, raw honey and wheatgerm oil. I described how to make it on page 15. Just apply and cover with a cloth bandage and change at least once a day. It should heal very quickly. You can also use the Green salve mentioned earlier as well. Either works well.

Another wonderful salve that works very well is from a combination of Myrrh and Goldenseal. This is extremely anti-bacterial and anti-viral. You can either make it up with equal parts of Myrrh and Golden seal mixed with olive oil and bees wax, similar to how I discussed how to make the Green salve or you can buy it from a company I have worked with for years. They are located at https://www.rawlife.com/black-herbal-salve/. Look for the product called Country Comfort Goldenseal-Myrrh Herbal Savvy. This is a marvelous salve that we have used on a large number of different skin conditions ranging from a simple scrape to cancer.

BRUISES:

Very common in childhood, they can also appear as bumps and bangs in adulthood, especially in those with a compromised circulatory system. While not necessarily a first aid moment, for some they can be embarrassing and unsightly.

HERBAL AIDS:

Plantain shines here again as a simple cure for bruises. Make a fomentation as described earlier or apply with the Green salve which has Plantain in it.

The Comfrey paste discussed above will also help diminish a bruise quite quickly.

CHAPTER 3

INTERMEDIATE FIRST-AID

Within this chapter I will discuss the next level of emergencies we could face without the help of a qualified health care provider. I will cover how to treat ear infections, eye injuries, minor dental mishaps, allergic reactions, minor bleeding and infections.

As always, please seek help from a qualified health care provider in case of an cmergency outside of the scope of your experience.

3.1 Ear Infections

So often they will start with that little itch, a minor annoyance and then can quickly escalate into nights of no sleep and difficulty hearing. We often see it in babies rubbing their ears but children and adults are subject to it's tortures. Sometimes earaches are caused by infection, cold in the head, a blow to the side of the head, and many other causes.

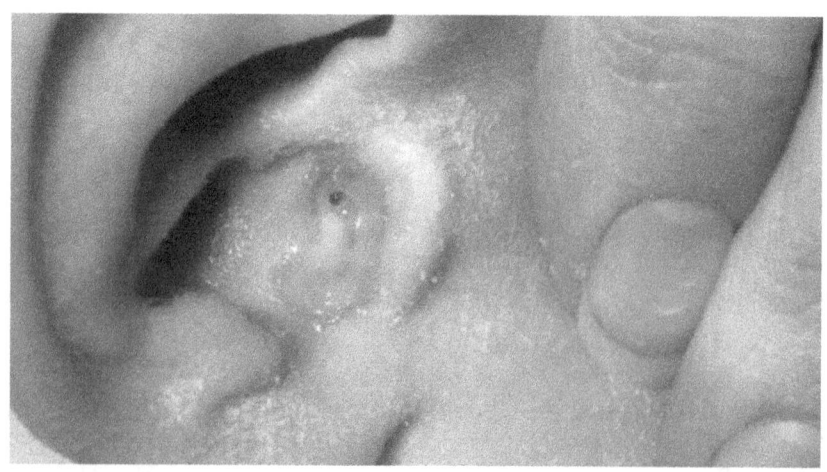

What is an ear infection?

An ear infection is an inflammation of the middle ear, usually caused by bacteria, that occurs when fluid builds up behind the eardrum. Anyone can get an ear infection, but children get them more often than adults. Five out of six children will have at least one ear infection by their third birthday. In fact, ear infections are the most common reason parents bring their child to a doctor. The scientific name for an ear infection is otitis media (OM). Adults can also get ear infections, but they are less common.

The infection usually affects the middle ear and is called otitis media. The tubes inside the ears become clogged with fluid and mucus. This can affect hearing, because sound cannot get through all that fluid.

If your child isn't old enough to say "My ear hurts," here are a few things to look for:

- Tugging at ears
- Crying more than usual
- Fluid draining from the ear
- Trouble sleeping
- Balance difficulties
- Hearing problems

What are the symptoms of an ear infection?

There are three main types of ear infections. Each has a different combination of symptoms.

- **Acute otitis media** (AOM) is the most common ear infection. Parts of the middle ear are infected and swollen and fluid is trapped behind the eardrum. This causes pain in the ear—commonly called an earache. Your child might also have a fever.
- **Otitis media with effusion** (OME) sometimes happens after an ear infection has run its course and fluid stays trapped behind the

eardrum. A child with OME may have no symptoms, but a doctor will be able to see the fluid behind the eardrum with a special instrument.
- **Chronic otitis media with effusion** (COME) happens when fluid remains in the middle ear for a long time or returns over and over again, even though there is no infection. COME makes it harder for children to fight new infections and also can affect their hearing.

In the clinic we have seen wonderful success with just a few simple remedies. Fortunately, nature provides a wonderful medicine cabinet full of natural "antibiotics" and anti-infectives.

HERBAL AIDS:

Garlic: Earache, inflammation of the middle ear, ear disease: Pack a small clove of garlic in gauze and place into the external ear passage; or drop 4-5 drops of Oil of Garlic into the ear channel, cover with flannel, and keep warm.

Mullein: Use warm mullein oil, 2-3 drops in the ear 2-3 times daily. Apple cider vinegar is also a healing agent.

Remember to always treat Both Ears: The simple, old-fashioned aids are sometimes very fast in giving relief. Always treat both ears, even if only one aches.

The lowly **onion** is also a powerful agent in healing. Lightly bake a large onion, cut it in half and while warm (not hot enough to irritate the area), bind one half of the onion over each ear. Bandage in place and hold bandage on with a nightcap, white skullcap, etc., and leave on all night

Dr. Christopher also has an amazing formula as a tincture which we have used very successfully over the years with our patients called the **Ear & Nerve Formula**: Dr. Christopher's Nervous System Formula with Black Cohosh: When this procedure is used as explained here, it can be helpful in promoting an improvement of poor equilibrium, failure of hearing, aiding the motor nerve, etc. With an eye dropper insert into each ear at night four to six drops of oil of garlic and four to six drops of the following herb tincture: blue Cohosh, Black cohosh, Blue vervain, Skullcap, and Lobelia, plugging ears overnight with cotton, six days a week, four to six months, or as needed. On the seventh day, flush ears with a small ear syringe using warm apple cider vinegar and distilled water half and half.

A few testimonials by Dr. Christopher.

1. **Garlic**: When my little girl had an earache I put a piece of fresh garlic in her ear and it was better by morning. The previous alternative was to go to the doctor and pay a lot of money for penicillin.

2. **Super Garlic Immune**: Dr. Christopher's Immune System Support Formula: The Super Garlic Immune formula contains Black Walnut. When Dr. Christopher was lecturing in Snowflake Arizona, he was describing the need for people to be prepared for the coming plagues in the last days.

Someone raised his hand and asked what should be used for the plague. Dr. Christopher, though he was a most noted herbalist, didn't have a ready answer! After a short prayer, he gave the Super Garlic Immune formula to the audience and then just forgot about it. Not long after, people began asking him for the formula again, as those at the Snowflake lecture had made it up and had, had marvelous results; they had cleared up flu, earache, eruptive diseases, car-sickness, and had even saved the life of a poisoned puppy! This Super Garlic Immune remedy is a most valuable combination.

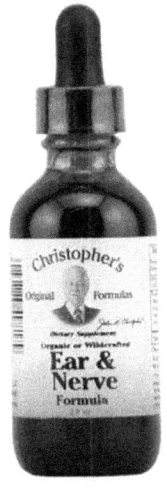

3.2 Dental

Here is a medical issue that can bring a grown man to his knees and not think twice about running to a dentist. There is little that is more painful or life disabling than a dental issue such as tooth infection or mouth sores. You cannot eat and it can even lead to heart issues in the future if not cared for properly. In the more severe cases you will be going to a dentist, but there are many times when it can be cared for successfully at home. Dr. Christopher was very successful with dental issues.

As stated by him: "Tooth problems start several generations back. The weakness of calcium deficiency is passed from parent to child. By following the same parental pattern of "poor food selection," each new crop of babies becomes weaker. "The sins (of omission and of commission) of the parents are passed on to the third and fourth generation." While the baby is being carried in the womb, Mother Nature is interested in that which is being produced more than the one producing. She is continually trying to upgrade humans and animals by drawing on the mother to supply the child. How often do we hear the expression, "Well, I'm carrying another child, that means more varicose veins and loss of more teeth - I don't see why mothers have to suffer this way." Please don't blame the Lord for these conditions, rather blame the use of pastries, soda pop, candy, sugar, ice cream, etc. The sugar leaches the calcium out of the body. Pregnancy is a strain on body calcium, because the mother must have enough calcium in her body for both her and the baby being formed, and later for nursing. If there is not enough calcium for her, because of this leaching process by the sugar (of past and present), the fetus draws on the mother's body. The calcium it now takes is from the bones, muscles, and the teeth, etc. Sometimes so much is taken from the mother that she will, after a number of babies, have bone and muscle problems from a great lack of calcium.

When a child is being formed and there is not enough calcium being supplied to the fetus, the jaw of the child will not form fully. It will be narrow instead of broad. When it is time for the child to cut teeth, they cannot come in "Straight" because of a crowded jaw space. So, naturally, they will come in crooked. Later as there is not enough room for the wisdom teeth, they must often be extracted before coming through. When the day comes that the jaw is adequately large and well-shaped to accommodate all thirty-two teeth without crowding them to crookedness, and the wisdom teeth can remain until old age (and in comfort), it will mean we humans have "gained enough wisdom" to keep them!

The basic cause of calcium loss, of course, as mentioned, is leaching out the calcium with sugars and a toxic body condition. Nearly all tooth decay comes from the blood stream, saliva, and the inside of the teeth, not only from the external surface. The teeth deteriorate but it is from the toxic blood stream and the enamel-destroying toxic saliva which is a result of an impure (toxic) blood stream. If a child has good wholesome food and has been given a "good solid start in life" with a full healthy set of teeth and jaws, he can go through life without tooth problems. The condition of perfect teeth is, of course, dependent upon a continual use of wholesome and proper foods."

One way to accomplish this level of calcium is to use a formula Dr. Christopher's created called **Calc-Tea**. Calc-Tea is made of Horsetail grass, Oat straw, Comfrey leaves and Lobelia. Horsetail grass and Oat straw are high in silica. Calcium can't be used in the body without the presence of Silica. The other Herbs support the function of the silica herbs in helping the body assimilate calcium.

> The formula is as follows:
> 6 parts Horsetail grass (Equisetum hyemale)
> 3 parts Oat straw (Avena sativa)
> 4 parts Comfrey root (Symphytum officinale)
> 1 part Lobelia (Lobelia inflata)

In this case a part is measured in weight, such as ounces. It can taken as a tea with one teaspoon to a cup of water or a tablespoon to a pint. It can also be taken in capsules.

The following testimonials attest to it's efficiency:

1. **Tooth Grows Back**: My oldest daughter age 13 now, had a dental cavity at age 7 (the only dental cavity among our six children). We had the cavity drilled out and a filling put in by our local dentist. Two years later, the filling

came out and a hole was left in her tooth. Nothing more was done about it except the herbal calcium formula that you recommend in your book, School of Natural Healing, made up of: Comfrey, horsetail, Oatstraw, and Lobelia. This combination of herbs has been used very consistently by the entire family over the last two years. We have recently discovered that the hole where the filling was is now completely grown over and is absolutely unnoticeable even under close inspection.

2. **Insomnia Cured**: I have found great relief by taking Dr. Christopher's calcium formula and thyroid formula through the night which was recommended in his "How Important is Calcium" newsletter. I have recommended this treatment to others and to my mother and they all have found it helps their insomnia also. -A.R., Williston, ND.

Sometimes the best defense is a good offense, preventative care. Dr. Christopher stated: "**Children need calcium if bones and teeth are to grow strong and well-formed. Adults need an adequate amount of calcium every day. During periods of pregnancy and lactation, women require much more calcium than normally, as they must also furnish extra calcium for the baby.** "

Another wonderful formula is Dr. Christopher's Herbal Tooth Powder. It can be purchased online or you can make it yourself. It is very easy to make and it is used instead of tooth paste for regularly brushing of your teeth. It is all I have used for years, brushing daily. The formula is as follows:

3 part Oak bark (Quercus alba)
6 parts Comfrey root (Symphytum officinale)
3 parts Horsetail grass (Equisetum hymale)
1 part Lobelia (Lobelia inflata)
1 part Cloves (Syzgyium aromaticum
3 parts Peppermint (Mnetha piperita)

A nice testimonial for the above tooth powder formula: **No Root Canal**: After breaking a tooth from biting my fingernails, I had to have a crown put on one of my bottom front teeth. This tooth aches all the time. Sometimes it's from the weather, sometimes from eating something, and sometimes from headaches. My tooth was so sensitive I couldn't eat corn on the cob!

When I complained about the pain, my dentist told me that if it keeps bothering me we might have to do a root canal. I started using Dr. Christopher's Herbal Tooth Powder to brush my teeth once or twice a week. As long as I remember to brush with the tooth powder, my tooth doesn't hurt. Whenever I forget to use it, my tooth starts to hurt again. I love the tooth powder, because it helped me avoid a root canal.

HERBAL AIDS:

For tooth pain use Clove oil or Plantain powder on the tooth at the roots.

An excellent treatment with a great history for gum disease and even cavities and blackened teeth uses the above tooth powder along with a Black walnut tincture. Each day, three times a day, brush your teeth with the above tooth powder. When you have finished brushing and have spit out the water now mix in a quarter cup of water with two dropper fulls of the Black walnut tincture. Swish this in your mouth for at least a minute and then swallow it. Do this at this dosage and rate for two weeks. If the gums are improving and the pain is gone you can drop the dosage to one dropper full a day.

I have also seen wonderful success with olive oil pulling. I have heard of others using coconut oil but I believe olive oil is more effective. We use this to aid in drawing out the infection from the teeth and gums. Swish it in your mouth at least three times a day during a serious infection. Hold it in the mouth for at least 10 minutes and then spit it out.

You can also use castor oil packs over an abscess in cases of severe infections or cysts caused by the infections. To do this soak a white cotton cloth in castor oil and place it over the cheek's skin nearest the infection or tooth pain. Now cover the cloth with a saran wrap and then place a towel over the wrap. Next, place a heating pad over the towel Do this as many times a day as you can, at least twice a day. I have seen serious cysts and infection begin to drain in just a couple of days. It may take weeks for the cyst to completely disappear.

3.3 Infections

Hospital-acquired infections with *Staphylococcus aureus*, especially methicillin-resistant *S. aureus* (MRSA) infections, are a major cause of illness and death and impose serious economic costs on patients and hospitals. Nosocomial (hospital acquired infection) bloodstream infections are a leading cause of death in the United States. If we assume a nosocomial infection rate of 5%, of which 10% are bloodstream infections, and an attributable mortality rate of 15%, bloodstream infections would represent the eighth leading cause of death in the United States.

Among the most common types of these infections include MRSA, septicemia and influenza and pneumonia. Infections can be either or both of a bacterial or viral nature. Unfortunately, as the rate in increase of MRSA proves, the bacteria soldiers are winning battle as they become more and more resistant to antibiotics.

The Threat of Antibiotic Resistance

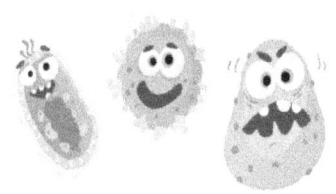

Increase in antibiotic resistance means that the effectiveness of antibiotics used to treat infections is diminished or non-existent.

"The use of antibiotics is the single most important factor leading to antibiotic resistance around the world."

2 Million the number of people in the US that acquire serious antibiotic-resistant infections each year

23,000 the number of people in the US that die as a direct result of antibiotic resistant infections each year

250,000 the number of people in the US that require hospital care for Clostridium difficil *(C. difficile: a unique bacterial infection directly related to antibiotic use and resistance)* infections each year

14,000 the number of people in the US that die from C. difficil infections each year

One of the most commonly prescribed drugs in the United States are antibiotics. According to the CDC:

- 50% of prescribed antibiotics are not needed or are not optimally effective as prescribed.
- 1 out 5 emergency visits are for adverse drug events involving antibiotics.
- $35 billion a year lost to productivity because of antibiotic usage.
- $20 billion estimated yearly excess in direct healthcare costs in part due to prolonged and/or costlier treatments.
- Individuals with an already compromised immune system are made worse by the use of antibiotics.
- At least 70% of Americans have a candida overgrowth due to the use of antibiotics, thereby compromising their immune systems further.

So, what can we do when we are threatened with an infection when going to the hospital has become such a possibly risky trip? The plant kingdom has a wide variety of medicines used successfully throughout history.

HERBAL AIDS:

By far, the best natural antibiotic or anti-infective we have used is hands down, the Stinking Rose, also known as the simple **Garlic**. It is a medical fact that three to five cloves of garlic is the equivalent in efficacy to an adult dose of penicillin, without destroying your gut micro-flora.

Garlic can be used in many ways but it CANNOT be cooked if you want any medicinal value out of it. It has approximately 35 sulfur compounds in it and this makes it such an effective antibiotic and the good news is that even If you are allergic to sulfur types of antibiotics, this one will not hurt you. But this is the reason it cannot be cooked as the compounds are destroyed with heat.

It can be dried and used in capsules. It can also be used in oils. A garlic oil compound is very effective for ear infections and such. To make a garlic oil simply chop up some garlic and put into a bottle and cover completely with olive oil. Shake for three days and then filter out the garlic pieces. That's it. Use the oil as needed.

Health Benefits of Garlic

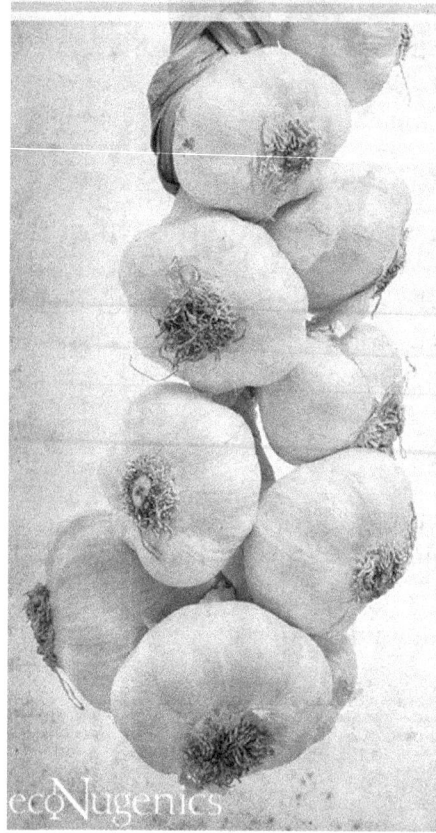

- Boosts Immune System
- Treats Athlete's Food
- Stops Toothaches
- Curbs Cold + Flu Effects
- Lowers Cholesterol
- Treat Insect Bites
- Promote Heart Health
- Clears Nasal Congestion
- Heal Cold Sores
- Kills Parasites
- Lowers Blood Pressure
- Repel Mosquitoes
- Prevent Blood Clots
- Aid Poor Digestion

Another great way to use garlic is as a paste. Please keep in mind that fresh garlic juice can actually burn the skin and this is why it needs to be in an oil or some other kind of salve or paste.

To make as a paste chop up several cloves of garlic and mix with petroleum jelly. This is the only time you will see me recommended this medium but it is basically inert and will hold the garlic while protecting the skin. If someone is ill with an infection or a cold or the flu you can make this paste and place on the bottoms of their bare feet. Cover with a cloth bandage and then their socks. Let them wear it all night. It is interesting to note how quickly garlic can pass into the system. You can place this paste on the feet and in a very short time you will be able to smell it on their breath.

Please remember, the fresher the garlic, the better.
As capsules take 3 or more capsules five times a day internally during an illness or infection.

OTHER HERBAL AIDS:

There are a number of herbs that also work very well for infections.

Onion poultice: This is an old but tried and true practice that has worked wonderfully for respiratory issues such as colds, the flu, bronchitis and even pneumonia. It involves the little cousin to garlic … the onion.

To make the poultice, take a white or yellow onion and chop up thoroughly. Place in the oven at about 250 to 300 degrees for about twenty minutes. You will know when it is done as the pieces are just starting to get "slimy". Now take them out and let them cool enough where they will not damage the skin and place over the chest while the patient is lying down. If this is for a baby then please make sure to rub some olive oil on the skin first to protect it as they are more sensitive than older children or adults.

Now cover the onions with a towel and then a heating pad. Keep on for at least a half an hour. Do this several times a day.

Onion cough syrup: You can also make the onions into an excellent cough syrup. Take a white or yellow onion and chop up and place into a sauce pan. Cover with raw honey and simmer over low heat for about 25 to 30 minutes. Strain and use the honey as a teaspoon to a tablespoon as needed for coughs.

Golden seal is a wonderful anti-viral. For colds and the flu, use three capsules five times a day until the patient is cured.

Echinacea – This herb works wonderfully as it fools the body into believing it was poisoned (though it was not). It causes the immune system to go into high gear. The problem is that after about five days the body realizes it is not being poisoned and will stop working. Take a break for a few days and start back up and the body will have forgotten and will ramp the immune system back up. Take two to three capsules five times a day during an infection or illness. This herb also works very well with Goldenseal.

Coconut oil is very effective when used topically on MRSA skin infections.

Cats Claw – This is an amazing herb for fighting bacteria, second to garlic. I use it when treating Lyme disease and it is very effective in killing the bacteria. Take two capsules five times a day during an illness.

For wound and skin infections please remember to use the **Herbadyne** mentioned in a previous section. Apply topically several times a day during the active part of the infection.

Another formula that has worked very well in the field is Dr. Christopher's **Infection Formula**. I have used it successfully for parasites, bacterial and viral infection and mold type illnesses.

The formula is as follows:

INFECTION FORMULA:

4 parts Plantain (Plantago major)
4 parts Black walnut (Juglans nigra)
4 parts Goldenseal root (Hydransis Canadensis)
2 parts Bugle weed (Lycopus virginicus)
1 part Marshmallow root (Althaea officinalis)
1 part Lobelia (Lobelia inflata)

All parts are measured in weight, for example one part equals one ounce.

During an infection, cold, the flu, etc., you take three capsules five times a day or if it is very serious you can use three to five capsules every hour until the patient improves and then you can drop the dosage to five times a day.

3.4 Allergic reactions

Food allergies are a growing epidemic in the United States with a diagnosis of anaphylactic food reactions increasing by 377 percent from 2007 to 2016. Peanuts are at the top with eggs and sea food coming in second and third. As the diet and quality of food in this nation continues to degrade these types of issues are becoming more common place in American households. The reactions can appear very mild from a simple case of hives and watery eyes and sniffles to a life threatening condition requiring immediate medical intervention, anaphylactic shock.

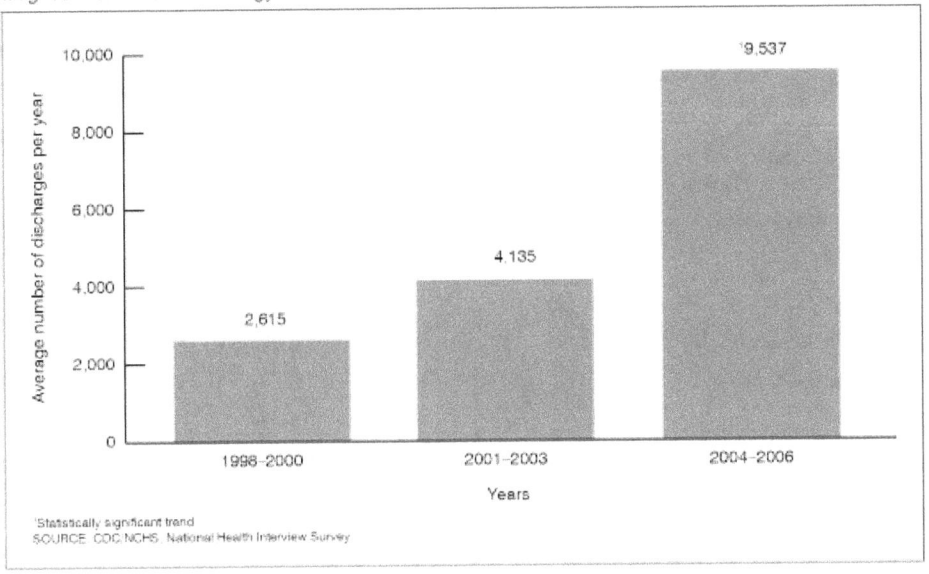

Figure 4. Average number of hospital discharges per year among children under age 18 years with any diagnosis related to food allergy: United States, 1998-2006

According to JAMA, the Journal for the American Medical Association: **The overall economic cost of food allergy was estimated at $24.8 (95% CI, $20.6-$29.4) billion annually ($4184 per year per child). Direct medical** costs were $4.3 (95% CI, $2.8-$6.3) billion annually, including clinician visits, emergency department visits, and hospitalizations. Costs borne by the family totaled $20.5 billion annually, including lost labor productivity, out-of-pocket, and opportunity costs. Lost labor productivity costs totaled $0.77 (95% CI, $0.53-$1.0) billion annually, accounting for caregiver time off work for medical visits. Out-of-pocket costs were $5.5 (95% CI, $4.7-$6.4) billion annually, with 31% stemming from the cost of special foods. Opportunity costs totaled $14.2 (95% CI, $10.5-$18.4) billion annually, relating to a caregiver needing to leave or change jobs.

The current standard treatments today utilizes a series of drugs aimed at suppressing the immune system. These include antihistamines and steroids. For severe allergic reactions the EpiPen is the choice for many. Unfortunately, it's cost has more the quadrupled n the last few years putting it outside of most patient's budgets when they have no insurance.

In this section I will go over a wide range of holistic, herbal medications you can do at home for treating anything from the mild watery eyes to the more severe anaphylactic shock. Always remember to seek a qualified healthcare provider in cases of emergency.

HERBAL AIDS:

Stinging Nettle: This wonderful little plant actually has very similar properties to Benadryl. It acts as an antihistamine, relieving the mild allergic reaction such as hive, watery eyes and sniffles without making you sleepy like Benadryl. We use it as an alcohol based tincture. During a mild allergic event such as seasonal allergies, we usually recommend two dropper fulls three times a day. You can also use it as needed and so you can use it throughout the day during a more severe hay fever attack, for example. It is non-toxic and therefore you will not overdose on it.

Immucalm: This formula was created by Dr. Christopher for calming the immune system while still allowing it to be strong. It is NOT an immune-suppressant and therefore will not leave you open to other infections, such as some of the other drugs can do. It is made from two herbs; Astragalus and

Marshmallow root. It can be purchased online or you can make it yourself at home. It also comes in a gentle glycerin based liquid formula for children.

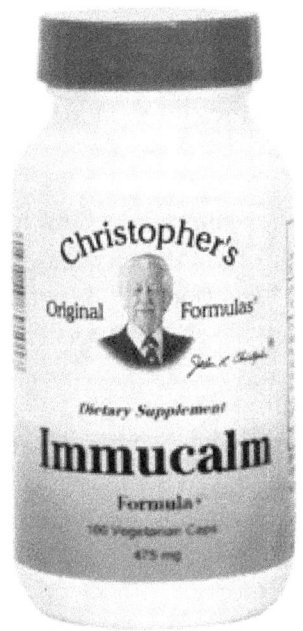
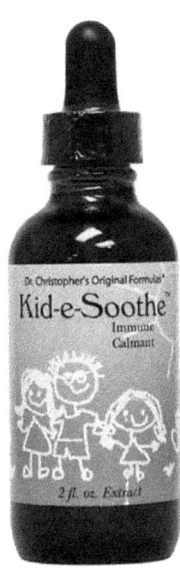

It is very simple to make it yourself. It is equal parts Astragalus and Marshmallow root. This has been used successfully with such issues as hayfever, allergy related asthma, Rheumatoid Arthritis, any auto-immune disease, and any type of hyper-immune disorder.

The above two formulas, Kid-e-Soothe and Stinging Nettle also can play an important part in dealing with anaphylactic shock where an EpiPen is not available. This happened once with a patient who could not afford to pay for the new costs of EpiPens and asked for a natural alternative. I informed her that such an issue is a medical emergency and she needed to be careful about her medical choices. She went ahead and requested the protocol.

This protocol requires having a full and sealed bottle of each of the two medications, Kid-e-Soothe and Stinging Nettle. She was to keep both with her at all times, just like she would with an EpiPen. She was very allergic to insect stings and bites such as a bee and had a history of life threatening reactions. If she were stung or bitten she was to IMMEDIATELY open both bottles and drink them completely as quickly as she could.

Well, it happened. She and a friend were sitting at poolside one day and she suddenly felt the bite on the top of her head. Her friend had been taught what to do and immediately got her friend's purse and cracked open both bottles and had her drink them immediately. She did so and they waited. Nothing happened.

After a few minutes her friend told her she would be in the house washing the dishes but would be watching from the kitchen window. The patient told her she felt fine and to go ahead. After about 20 minutes her friend noted that she seemed to be slumping somewhat in the poolside chair. She ran out to see if she was alright.

The patient, not used to alcohol from the Stinging Nettle, informed her friend she was feeling great but was a bit looped. All was well and she immediately purchased another set of the herbal medications.

OTHER USEFUL AIDS FOR ALLERGIES:

Apple cider Vinegar: Braggs Apple Cider Vinegar is supposed to work well with allergies due to it's ability to cut mucous production and cleanse the lymphatic system. During allergy season just mix a tablespoon or two in a glass of distilled water and drink three times a day.

Neti Pot: For those familiar with it, it is simply a spouted container, similar to a little teapot. You fill it with distilled water and a quarter teaspoon of salt. You use this to rinse out your sinus cavity. Use a pre-made saline rinse or make your own by dissolving 1/4 teaspoon of Himalayan or just plain sea salt in a quart of boiled distilled water. Cool completely. Put in the Neti Pot and pour through one nostril and let it drain out the other. Make sure to do both nostrils.

Raw Local Honey: Raw, local honey from a compassionate bee keeper works very well as it contains pollen from your area. Taking a tablespoon a day all year is like giving yourself a gentle vaccine. The theory is that it gradually and safely builds up an immunity to the pollen and you experience little to no seasonal allergy issues after.

Mullein and Lobelia Tincture: Sometimes during an allergy attack, breathing may become difficult. In lieu of having a rescue inhaler we like to use what was very common among the Native Americans. This utilized the herb called Mullein, a very common plant in the United States. It was well known by them to use it during an asthmatic attack. They would breath in the smoke of the leaves and the attack would stop immediately.

We make it into a tincture of 3 parts Mullein and 1 part Lobelia. We instruct our patients to use a dropper full on the tongue as needed to stop the asthma attack.

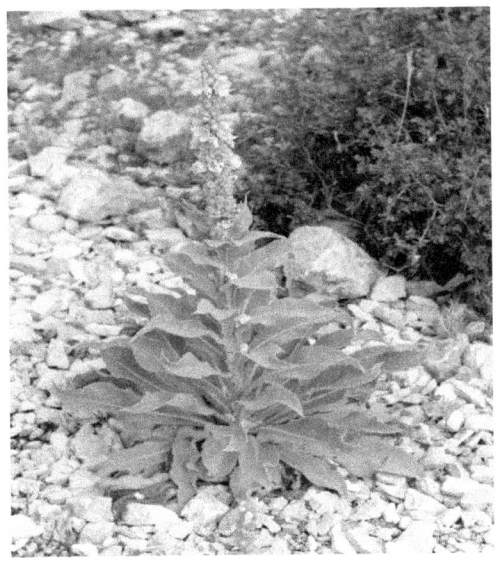

Mullein

Gut Health: As described in my book *A Complete Body Repair, Healing Candida, Parasites and Heavy Metal Toxicity Naturally*, I discuss the importance of a healthy micro-flora colony in the gut. This is 70 to 80% of your immune system and this is a leading cause of allergies as an unhealthy environment can lead to "Leaky Gut Syndrome". I have seen MANY patients lose their allergies when the gut health was restored to a normal condition. I myself used to be very allergic to Poison Oak but no longer experience it once I healed my intestinal environment.

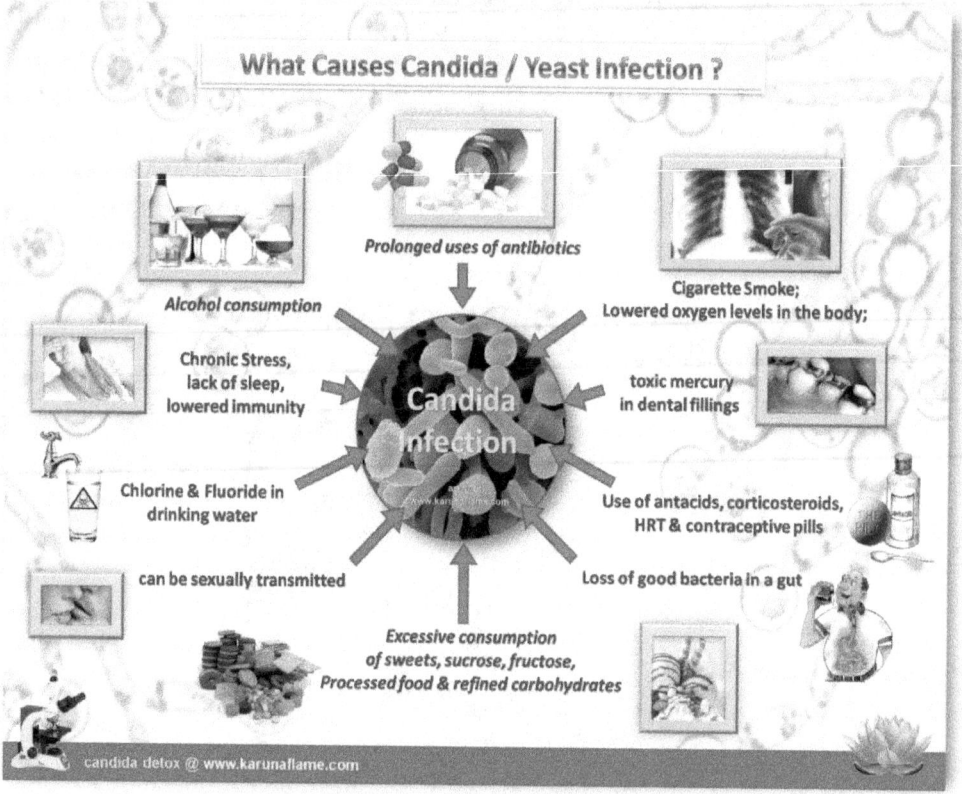

3.5 Bleeding - Minor

One of the most frightening things you can experience at home is an accident with resulting bleeding. As defined by The School of Natural Healing: The escaping of blood internally or externally. Blood coughed from the lungs is generally of a bright red color and is usually mixed with sputum. The problem is often preceded by nausea and stomach disorder with blood passing through the bowels. Simple enough. What do we do about minor events?

This section deals mainly with minor bleeding issues along the lines of cuts, scrapes, nose bleeds and mouth issues. Chapter four will focus more on the very serious bleeding problems, external, internal, during labor and such.

HERBAL AIDS:

Cayenne: By far, I know of NO better styptic than the sizzling cayenne. I have seen miracles with the use of this herb. Dr. Christopher would often remark how you could count to 60 after using this herb and you would often see the bleeding stopped before you reached the end. I have personally seen this happen.

Cayenne is known as a rubefacient. This means that where ever cayenne touches it brings blood to that area. While there are many benefits this brings, for example, bringing more oxygen and nutrients, what we see in this case is an equalization of blood pressure. It simply pulls the pressure off of the wound and slows or stops the bleeding.

In the case of an open wound or nose bleed, simply put a few drops of cayenne tincture on your tongue. You can also use pure cayenne powder as it will work as well. If you are brave, you can also put a small amount of the cayenne into the wound. Yes, it will be very hot but it can stop the bleeding very quickly. Once done, simply count to 60 and watch the results.

My wife is a wonderful example of this. On two separate instances, within a week of each other, provided wonderful proof to cayenne's effectiveness. The first incident involved a mandolin while slicing up zucchini for me. She was slicing the zucchini and grew impatient and removed the blade guard. It was the next slice that removed a small portion of her thumb. Blood began to spurt out of the wound with each heartbeat. Fortunately, she had some holistic first aid training prior to this and immediately grabbed the cayenne tincture we keep on hand for just such emergencies.

She immediately poured some of the cayenne tincture on the counter and rubbed her open wound in it! Needless to say, it was quite hot and painful. The good news is that cayenne causes zero tissue damage, even if it feels as though it is. She also squirted a dropper full in her mouth and then began to count. By the time she hit sixty there was barely an ooze from her open cut.

Well, another incident occurred about a week later. She had finished washing the dishes and they were drying in the dish drainer. When it came to time to put them away, she reached and grabbed a handful of silverware to put in the draw right next to her. In the middle of the handful was a knife pointing down. She relaxed her grip slightly and down went the knife, straight into the top of her foot. She looked down to see a knife standing straight up, embedded in the top of her foot. She is a tough Alabama, Cherokee woman and she knew what to do. She simply reached down and pulled out the knife. Of course, out came the blood. Fortunately, she still had the bottle of cayenne tincture on the counter. She chose this time to not put it straight into the wound but squirted a dropper full into her mouth. Again, she counted. After sixty seconds, the bleeding had completely stopped. A wonderful miracle cayenne is for any home first-aid kit.

HOW TO MAKE CAYENNE TINCTURE:

Making cayenne tincture is a simple process, and the only drawback to making your own is the time spent waiting for the tincture to be ready to use. Cayenne tincture can be made from dried cayenne peppers or cayenne pepper powder.

Pack a 1-quart jar tightly with cayenne peppers. If using whole peppers, make sure to chop them thoroughly to increase surface exposure to the alcohol. If using cayenne pepper powder, fill the jar half-full.

Fill the jar with vodka to within a half-inch of the jar's top. Use apple cider vinegar or glycerin if you don't want to use alcohol.

Place the lid on the jar and tighten.

Store in a cool, dark place for two weeks, making sure to walk by at least once a day and shake vigorously.

Drain the tincture though cheesecloth to remove the peppers from the liquid.

Pour the strained tincture into smaller, colored bottles and cap. Be sure to label the bottles. The tincture will keep indefinitely in a cool area.

Dr. Christopher had wonderful advice for those who suffer with chronic nosebleeds:

Nosebleeds: Unless it is from injury, nosebleed results from a calcium deficiency. It is caused by the rupture of a small vessel in the nose due to pressure in the head. There are many causes for nosebleeds, but the weakness stems from calcium deficiency. Of course, it does not matter how much calcium is in the body if one is hit in the nose with a good blow; bleeding will start. A teaspoon of cayenne in a cup of water (hot preferred) taken internally will stop most nosebleeds quickly. In an emergency such as this we use cayenne. As mentioned a teaspoon of cayenne pepper in a glass of water and drunk right down will stop a nosebleed in nearly every instance, by the time you can count to ten. This is not a miracle; it is the principle of the cell stimulant cayenne traveling through the entire blood stream and regulating the pressure so the pressure of the flow is the same in the feet as in the head or any other part of the body. This takes the heavy pressure off the hemorrhaging area and allowing a quick coagulation. One of our very finest herbal foods is our calcium formula [Herbal Calcium Formula] of four parts Comfrey root, six parts horsetail grass, three parts oat straw and one part Lobelia. Make this into a tea, using a cup (one teaspoon of combined herbs to cup of distilled water) morning and one evening or two or three capsules or tablets two or three times in a day.

Stinging Nettle: In Russia, it is used as a valued antiseptic and astringent. The pulverized dry herb is sniffed to stop nose bleeding.

OTHER HERBAL AIDS:

Shepard's Purse: What a gentle little herb shaped like a heart. There is an ancient theory called the Doctrine of Signatures where it states that plants of a particular shape heals in the body similar. I can see that with this little herb with it's shape and the circulatory system.

As stated by Dr. Christopher: "Most herbalists agree on most of the medicinal qualities of Shepherd's Purse, they being astringent, styptic, diuretic, anti-scorbutic, vasoconstrictor and blood coagulant, which therefore makes it anti-hemorrhagic (or hemostatic). Additionally, Kloss listed it as having detergent and vulnerary qualities.

Grieve said it was anti-diarrheal, Duke mentioned its antioxidant qualities and Schwartz claimed it to be anti-inflammatory. Moore got more specific, mentioning that Shepherd's Purse uses were: "Urinary tract astringent, uric acid diuretic for hyperuricemia; hemostatic for hematuria, excess menses, and so forth; and an oxytocin agonist for postpartum bleeding or difficult placenta delivery."

DOSAGE: For bleeding issues take a teaspoon of the tincture every few minutes or a half a cup every ten minutes until bleeding stops.

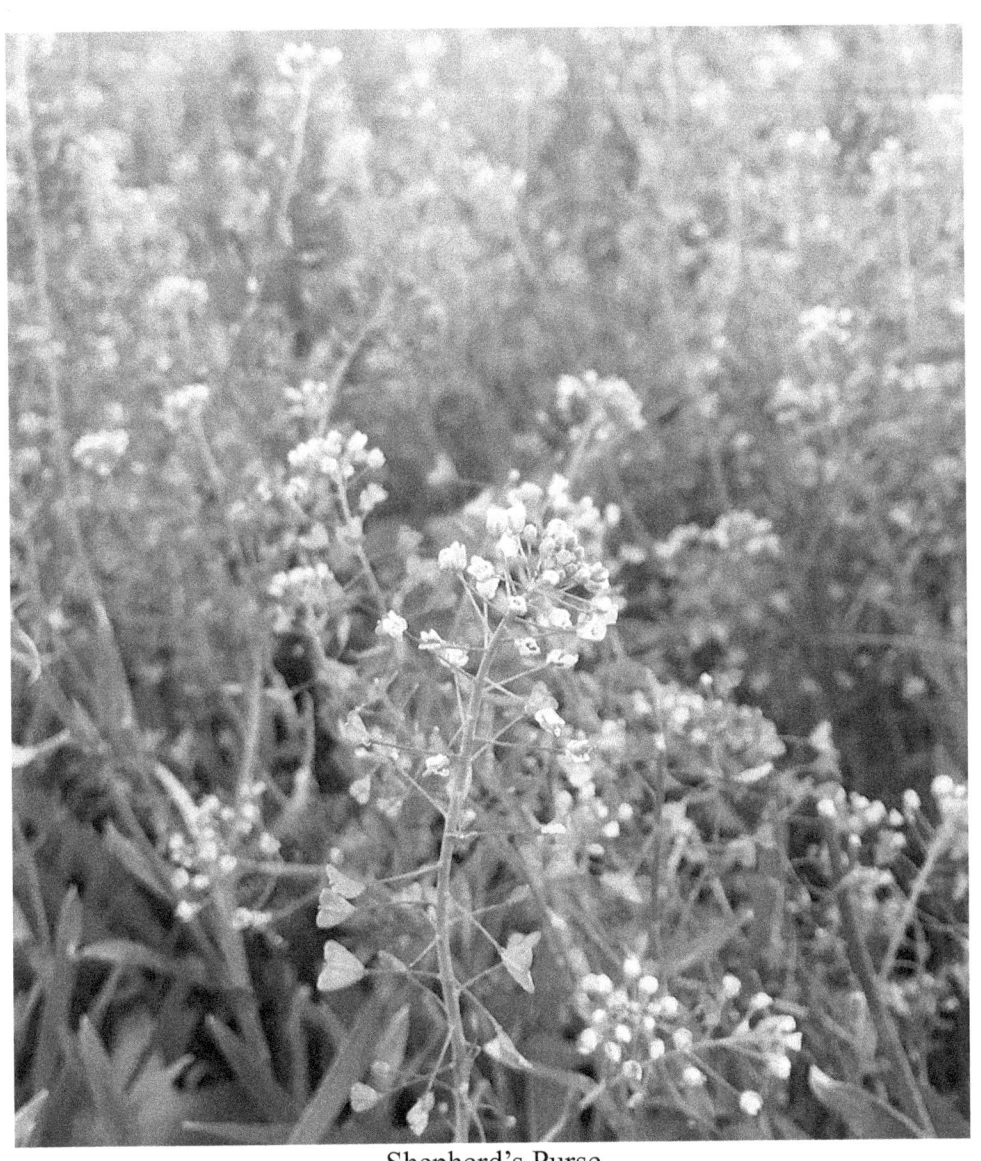
Shepherd's Purse

3.6 Eye injuries and infections

Of all of the senses, I believe the most debilitating in the short term would have to be eyesight. This section will be dealing with any problem affecting the eyes in a first aid type event such as infections, injuries, and conjunctivitis.

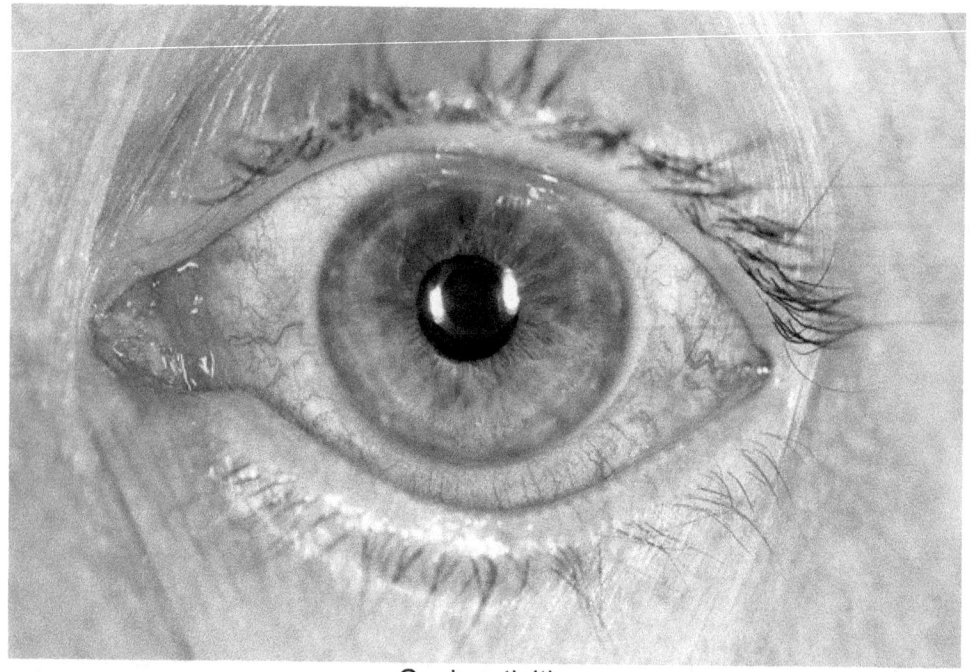

Conjunctivitis

CONJUNCTIVITIS: Also known as pink-eye, this is an infection, usually bacterial, and an inflammation of the conjunctiva. The conjunctiva is the thin clear tissue that lies over the white part of the eye and lines the inside of the eyelid. Children are usually the largest group who are afflicted with this infection.

Several things could be to blame, including:

- Viruses, including the kind that causes the common cold
- Bacteria
- Irritants such as shampoos, dirt, smoke, and pool chlorine
- A reaction to eyedrops
- An allergic reaction to things like pollen, dust, or smoke. Or it could be due to a special type of allergy that affects some people who wear contact lenses.
- Fungi, amoebas, and parasites

For an herbalist, this can be a very easy condition to treat. We prefer this to the use of antibiotics since they will usually destroy the micro-flora in the intestinal tract, thereby suppressing the body's immune system.

HERBAL AIDS FOR CONJUNCTIVITIS AND OTHER INFECTIONS:

Red Raspberry tea: A simple eyewash can be made from this tea and dripped into the eye when cooled. You can also use the cooled teabag after you have made tea with it and place it over the closed eye for about a half an hour, several times a day.

Raw Honey: Raw honey from a compassionate bee keeper is very antibiotic in nature. They have actually taken honey out of pyramids, laid down over two thousands years ago and was still viable. Take a drop of the honey and place into the eye and ask the patient to blink several times. It may take a couple of times a day but the results are amazing.

Mother's milk: Yes, I said mother's milk, human mother's milk. It is very high in natural antibiotics and can clear up a case of pink-eye over night. Use the same as the raw honey described above.

Dr. Christopher's Herbal Eyebright: As stated by Dr. Christopher: "this formula is excellent for helping to brighten and heal the eyes, and it is known to help remove the cataracts and heavy film from the eyes. "I personally have seen patients who needed to wear glasses and were able to give them up after a couple of month of using this eyewash regularly. It is made from bayberry, cayenne, eyebright, golden seal and red raspberry leaves. The formula is as follows or you can purchase it online:

1 part Bayberry bark (Myrica cerifera)
1 part Eyebright (Euphrasia officinalis)
1 part Golden seal root (Hydrastis canadensis)
1 part Red Raspberry leaves (Rubus idaeus)
1/8 part cayenne (Capsicum annuum)

It can be drank as a tea, 1cup twice a day along with using as an eyewash.

To use as an eyewash:
Start each morning by filling up a glass eye cup about two thirds with clean distilled water. Place one drop of the Herbal Eyebright tincture into it. At first it will sting a little so we ask that you start slowly. Now, move the eye cup over the eye socket and tip your head back. Some may spill out so you can do this in the shower or place a towel over you neck for any leakage. Open you eye and look around like you would under water for about 30 to 60 seconds. Now repeat for the other eye but first wash the cup out and start over. This way you lower the risk of passing back and forth bacteria. Do this both in the morning and at night before bed. You can also drink a cup of the tea each time.

As the days or week go by, increase the dosage all the way up to about five drops or more. Again, we have seen wonderful results doing this procedure.

For all of the above protocols: follow until the issue is resolved.

All of the above herbal remedies also work on stys.

Baby Clogged Eye Duct: If your baby has an eye infection which is not gonorrheal you can suspect a plugged tear duct. Many mothers gently massage the area and/or wash it with eyebright and golden seal tea, which sometimes helps open the duct. If it doesn't open after a couple of months, you may wish to go to a good eye doctor for surgical opening of the duct.

Foreign Particles: If you get a foreign particle in your eye, or if your eyes become red and irritated, you can wash them either with Dr. Christopher's Eyewash, being sure to strain the tea carefully through a fine, clean cotton cloth, or a simple tea of red raspberry leaves. These teas help astringe and heal the irritated surface.

Some testimonials from Dr. Christopher and my practice:

1.) **Subretinal Hemorrhage**: My right eye went bad last January, diagnosed as "subretinal hemorrhage" which left me with probably 20-30% vision. Since using Eyebright Comb. [Herbal Eyebright], I now have 70 or 80% vision. Miracle Medicines-God's wonderful herbs.

2.) **Eye Pain**: The eyebright combination [Herbal Eyebright] has brought good results for a very severe pain behind one eye. (I have had this for over two years and the doctors have been unable to find the cause).

3.) In my practice I had a gentleman come in to the clinic complaining of having a restriction on his drivers license requiring him to wear eyeglasses. He used the Herbal eyewash formula for 60 days. When he returned to the DMV he was retested and passed the eye exam. The restriction was removed from his license.

4.) A mother brought her ten year old girl into the clinic one day with a very serious case of pink-eye. The school had sent her home. After using the eyewash for just a couple of days, the eye had healed enough where she was able to go back to school.

CHAPTER 4

ADVANCED FIRST-AID

4.1 Major Bleeding/Shock/Deep Cuts and Wounds

In the previous chapter we discussed coping with bleeding injuries, mainly minor and external. In this section we will cover how to treat more serious injuries such as internal, bleeding during labor and more serious external wounds when the opportunity for emergency medical care is not available.

When coping with a significant injury resulting in high blood loss shock is a very significant possibility and this along can kill a patient. It is important that we know the signs of shock and how to treat them.

SHOCK : SIGNS & SYMPTOMS

- ✛ **Discolourisation of Face**
- ✛ **Loss of Power**
- ✛ **Slow/weak Pulse**
- ✛ **Cold Sweating**
- ✛ **Irregular Breathing/Shallow breathing**
- ✛ **Nausea & Giddiness**
- ✛ **Clammy & Sandy Skin**
- ✛ **Fall in Temperature**

According to the Mayo Clinic: Shock is a critical condition brought on by the sudden drop in blood flow through the body. Shock may result from trauma, heatstroke, blood loss, an allergic reaction, severe infection, poisoning, severe burns or other causes. When a person is in shock, his or her organs aren't getting enough blood or oxygen. If untreated, this can lead to permanent organ damage or even death.

Signs and symptoms of shock vary depending on circumstances and may include:

- Cool, clammy skin
- Pale or ashen skin
- Bluish tinge to lips or fingernails (or gray in the case of dark complexions)
- Rapid pulse
- Rapid breathing
- Nausea or vomiting
- Enlarged pupils
- Weakness or fatigue
- Dizziness or fainting
- Changes in mental status or behavior, such as anxiousness or agitation.

Treatment for shock needs to be immediate. Take the following steps:

- Lay the person down and elevate the legs and feet slightly, unless you think this may cause pain or further injury.
- Keep the person still and don't move him or her unless necessary.
- Begin CPR if the person shows no signs of life, such as not breathing, coughing or moving.
- Loosen tight clothing and, if needed, cover the person with a blanket to prevent chilling.
- Don't let the person eat or drink anything.
- If the person vomits or begins bleeding from the mouth, and no spinal injury is suspected, turn him or her onto a side to prevent choking.

HERBAL AIDS FOR SHOCK AND MAJOR BLEEDING:

Here again, we return to that miracle herb ... cayenne. It is useful for both shock and bleeding injuries. As quoted from Dr. Christopher: "General Instructions For Shock: When a person goes into shock, the administration of medicinal aids orally will often be difficult or impossible. In this case an anus injection (or enema) which will cause relaxation is applicable. Use one cup (to a pint maximum) of catnip, peppermint, skullcap, spearmint, or Valerian.

Massage the abdomen and parts of the spine with Lobelia externally and make sure that the patient gets undisturbed rest. Cayenne should be taken internally to help equalize the blood pressure and insure that the internal functions will remain stabilized during the intense systemal distress."

When shock is caused by hemorrhaging: "Hemorrhage throws many people into shock and can bring on death very rapidly. If the wound is small, the blood usually coagulates and the area seals itself, but if the rupture is large, some herbal aid is needed. The first thing one should think about is cayenne as quickly as possible. Using one teaspoon to the cup, as hot as can be taken without scalding. This will help stop any hemorrhage, internal or external, by the time a person can count to ten. If the rupture is external and cayenne is not available, Comfrey placed over the wound will stop bleeding quickly."

The **Bach Flower Rescue Remedy** also works very well for shock to aid the patient to quickly recover. Give a few drops at the time of the incident.

Cayenne for serious wounds: In wounds, though the wound is cut and exposed to the bone, that wound may be filled with cayenne pepper (and if cayenne is not available, black pepper) and it will heal beautifully and stop the bleeding. Many people, when they seen the skin ruddier by cayenne, believe that the skin is irritated; but cayenne is a counter-irritant; there is no itching involved with it. What cayenne is actually doing is bringing the blood to the surface to take away any toxic poisons, or to start the healing; so the redness comes to the skin from the blood that has rushed to the surface to assist in carrying off wastes

Aloe Vera: Other external uses for the herb include treatment for all kinds of wounds--scrapes, cuts, etc. The gel seems to mildly kill the germs on the surface and promote healing. The herb is high in calcium, which reduces bleeding with its coagulating action, at the same time helping to stimulate circulation of blood in the surrounding areas to bring oxygen to the surface.

Ulcers: We need to go to the cause of ulcers and eliminate those but we can begin by relieving the pain and healing the tissues. Cayenne pepper should be taken by the teaspoon (start with 1/4 tsp. three times a day and work up to 1 teaspoonful three times a day). The cayenne pepper will even cauterize a bleeding ulcer.

FOR TREATING WOUNDS AND ENCOURAGING HEALING:

Having covered chock and bleeding, what do we do about the actual healing of the wound? Again, these are suggestions for folks without access to a qualified healthcare provider.

I mentioned earlier about using holistic medications such as **Herbadyne** and the **Green Salve.** They both easily apply here but I would like to give a word of warning. I do not apply a healing salve too quickly to a deep, open wound. The salves we are discussing here are very fast acting and can cause a wound to seal very quickly. If the wound was not properly cleansed first and not had an antiseptic applied first than dirt and bacteria could get trapped in the closing wound.

The first thing of course is to stem the bleeding as shown above. Next, clean the wound thoroughly with water or Hydrogen Peroxide. It is at this point you can then liberally use something like our Herbadyne formula. It will most likely sting but it is doing it's job. I would not use a strong healing salve for at least a day, to give the wound a chance to clean out.

One of the best formulas I have worked with for quick wound healing is Dr. Christopher's B, F and C. You can make it into a salve, capsules, syrup, shampoo, oil, etc. It stands for Bone, Flesh and Cartilage and it is meant to heal each of those tissues very quickly. You can purchase it online or you can make it with the included formula here.

6 Parts Oak Bark (Quercus alba)
3 Parts Marshmallow Root (Althaea officinalis)
3 Parts Mullein Herb (Verbascum thapsus)
2 Parts Wormwood (Artemisia absinthium)
1 Part Lobelia (Lobelia inflata)
1 Part Skullcap (Scutellaria lateriflora)
6 Parts Comfrey Root (Symphytum officinalis)
3 Parts Walnut Bark or leaves (Juglans nigra)
3 Parts Gravel root (Eupatorium purpureum)

This combination has saved many, many lives and limbs. If you will look back at page 17 you will see the foot that was healed, in part, with this combination because of the Comfrey in it. I have seen cases where deep, serious wounds healed with no scarring afterwards.

For very serious wounds, I would take the B, F and C in both an oral and an external treatment. During the beginning of the healing process the usual dosage is 5 capsules five times a day until the worse is over. It can take days or weeks, depending on the severity of the wound. At the same time I would also apply the B, F and C as a salve to the wound, after a day or two of using something like the Herbadyne as an antiseptic. After a couple of days you can start using the B, F and C salve. Make sure to apply the Herbadyne or some other natural antiseptic first and then the salve on top of it. Bandage over the salve. Change the dressing and reapply the antiseptic and the salve each day.

DOGS LEGS SAVED:

I have also seen the above salve used on other animals such as dogs. In two separate cases, I have seen dogs destined by their vets to have a leg amputated due to gaping open wounds. On both occasions, the caregivers chose to use the B, F and C salves on them and the legs completely healed. Both vets were quite amazed at the results.

Testimonials from Dr. Christopher:

1.) Cayenne and the Gunshot Wound: Once a child was shot in the abdomen; a bullet hit the spine, ricocheted, and made a second wound leaving the body. One of Dr. Christopher's herbal students, living next door, heard the shot and raced over, as she knew that the parents were not home and that the children, ages eight and four, would not be shooting guns. There was the eight-year-old gushing blood out both sides. She ran to the cabinet and mixed a tablespoonful of cayenne in a glass of water; she poured it down the boy and immediately called the ambulance, which was eighteen miles away. The emergency room attendant said that the boy would probably bleed to death, being that the distance was so great.

The ambulance arrived and rushed the child (who had been playing "Cops and Robbers" with his father's pistol, which he had found under the pillow of the bed, to the Primary Children's Hospital eighteen miles away. When he arrived, he was the center of attraction, not because his case was so dangerous, but because he was chatting a mile a minute--and there was no bleeding. The bleeding had stopped by the time they arrived at the hospital. The chief doctor said to the parents, "I have seen many accident victims in my life, but this is the first time in such an emergency operation that I have opened an abdomen to find no blood, except for a small amount that was there before the bleeding stopped so quickly. This has saved your boy's life."

2.) Stomach Ulcer: I had symptoms of a stomach ulcer and I drank the Cayenne Pepper and now I have no more symptoms. Thank you again for your information on Cayenne and how it works for bleeding and heart attacks.

3.) Cayenne: A person in our audience told how he had cut deeply with a sharp instrument the inside of his hand, fingers and palm. The blood spurted out in streams. He poured a large amount of cayenne pepper into the wound, and within seconds the blood flow slowed down to congealed dripping and the bleeding stopped entirely before many seconds had passed. With a goodly amount of cayenne covering the wound, he then wrapped it. He was so excited about the rapid results he could hardly wait for the regular herb meeting. But, as he said, the "punch line" was lost, because instead of a nasty ragged scar to show how severely he had been hurt, the area was healed and there was no scar.

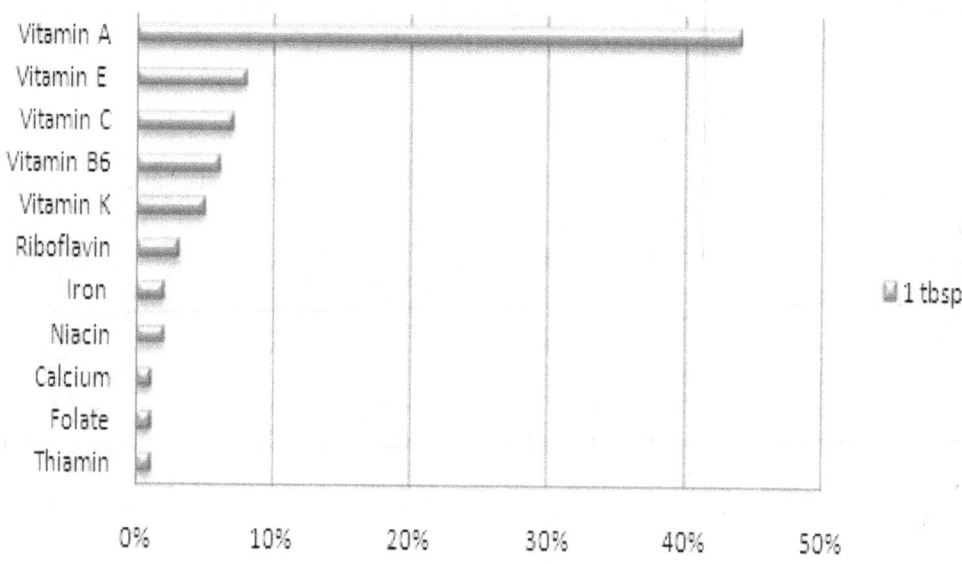

4.2 Poisoning

Unfortunately, this is an all too common occurrence in many households across America. In 2017, the 55 U.S. poison control centers provided telephone guidance for nearly 2.12 million human poison exposures.

	Year: 2017
Human Poison Exposures	2,115,186
Animal Poison Exposures	51,164
Confirmed Non-Exposures	5,523
Info Calls - Drug ID	96,221
Info Calls - Other	339,319
Total	2,607,413

According to poison.org: While young children (younger than 6 years) comprise a disproportionate percentage of the cases, poisoning affects ALL age groups, from infants to seniors. Peak poisoning frequency occurs in one and two year olds, but poisonings in teens and adults are more serious. Notice that the greater proportion of males in poison exposures occurring in children younger than 13 years switches to a female predominance in teens and adults.

Across all ages, there were 640 poison exposures reported per 100,000 population. The highest incidence occurred in one and two year olds (7,542 and 7,270 exposures/100,000 children in the respective age groups). For ages 50 years or older, 250 exposures were reported per 100,000 population.

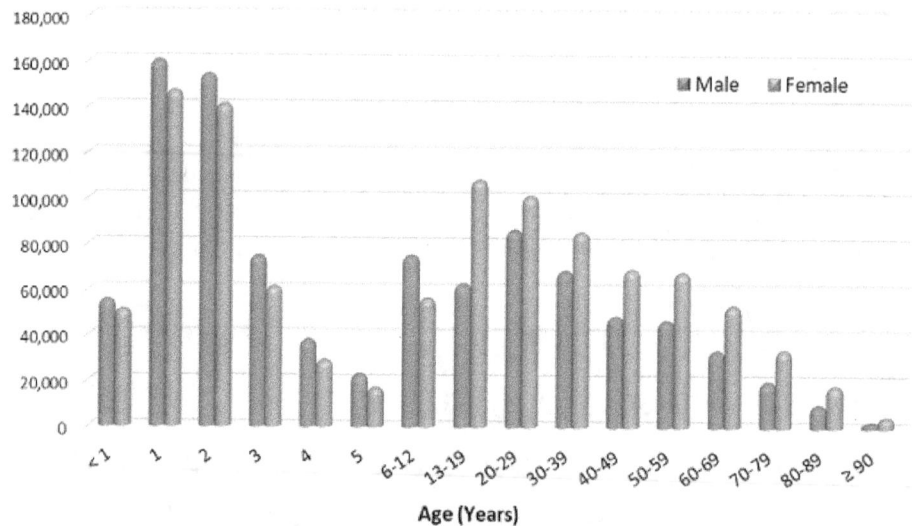

The most common substances involved in childhood poisonings reported:

- Cosmetics and Personal care products
- Cleaning substances
- Analgesics
- Foreign bodies/toys/Misc.
- Topical preparations
- Antihistamines
- Vitamins
- Pesticides
- Dietary supplements
- Plants

The most common substances involved in adult poisonings reported:

- Analgesics
- Sedative/Hypnotics/Anti-psychotics
- Antidepressants
- Cardiovascular drugs
- Household cleaning substances
- Alcohols
- Anticonvulsants

- Pesticides
- Stimulants and street drugs
- Antihistamines

What is also interesting is that the leading cause of children's poisoning in the 1990s was Flintstones vitamins with iron. They taste and look like candy so children were eating as such and the high iron content was poisoning them. I have in my practice treated children for iron toxicity from well meaning parents thinking if a little is good, more is better.

A significant number of poisonings are also due to heavy metal toxicity from such metals as lead. The scope of that subject is greater than a first aid treatment. If you would like to learn more about how to cure chronic heavy metal poisoning than please check out our book *A Complete Body Repair, Healing Candida, Parasite and Heavy Metal Toxicity Naturally*.

The type of first aid for poisoning varies depending on the type of chemical ingested. Overall, to start with, a very good rule of thumb is to not induce vomiting unless you have been instructed otherwise by a qualified healthcare provider. It used to a be standard decades ago to induce vomiting but it has been found that it can greatly increase the damage depending on the type of poison. So for now, no inducing your patient to vomit. We will work instead in strengthening the body's own defenses and neutralizing the poison.

Let's start with the basics. According to PSEP (Pesticide Safety Education Program):

Poison on the Skin
The sooner the poison is washed off the patient, the less the injury.

- Remove clothing and drench skin with water (shower, hose, faucet, pond, ditch).
- Cleanse skin and hair thoroughly with soap and water. (Don't abrade or injure the skin while washing.)
- Dry and wrap in a blanket

Warning: Do not allow any of the pesticide to get on you while you are helping the victim.

Chemical Burns of the Skin

- Remove contaminated clothing.
- Wash the skin with large quantities of cold running water.
- Immediately cover loosely with a clean, soft cloth.
- Avoid use of ointments, greases, powders, and other drugs in the first aid treatment of chemical burns.

Poison in the Eye

It is very important to wash the eye as quickly, but as gently, as possible.

- Hold eyelids open, wash eyes with a gentle stream of clean running water at body temperature.
- Continue washing for 15 minutes or more.
- Do not use chemicals or drugs in wash water. They may increase the extent of injury.

Inhaled Poisons (Dust, Vapors, Gases)

If victim is in an enclosed area use an air-supplied respirator to get to him.

- Carry patient (do not let him walk) to fresh air immediately.
- Open all doors and windows.
- Loosen all tight clothing.
- Apply artificial respiration if breathing has stopped or is irregular.
- Keep patient as quiet as possible.
- If patient is convulsing, watch his breathing and protect him from falling and striking his head. Pull his chin forward so his tongue does not block his air passage.
- Do not give alcohol in any form.

Swallowed Poisons

The most important decision you have to make when aiding a person who has swallowed a pesticide or poison is whether to induce vomiting or not.

The decision must be made quickly and accurately; the victim's life may depend on it. Usually it is best to get rid of the swallowed poison fast. But: **NEVER** induce vomiting if the victim is unconscious or is in convulsions. The victim could choke to death on vomitus.

Find out what poison has been ingested. **NEVER** induce vomiting if the victim has swallowed a corrosive poison. A corrosive poison is a strong acid or alkali (base) such as dinoseb (DN Compounds). The victim will complain of severe pain and have signs of severe mouth and throat burns. A corrosive poison wil burn the throat and mouth as severely coming up as it did going down.

Most labels on emulsifiable concentrate and solution formulations suggest the victim should not have vomiting induced. However, when the toxicity of the pesticide is marked, its removal may be essential.

Corrosive Poisons

The best first aid is to dilute the poison as quickly as possible. For acids or alkalis (bases), give the patient water or preferably a plant based milk - one (1) cup for victims under five (5) years; or one (1) to two (2) glasses for patients over five (5) years. The plant milk is better than water because it dilutes and helps neutralize the poison. Water only dilutes the poison.

It is very important that the victim get to a hospital without delay. **DO NOT INDUCE OR ENCOURAGE VOMITING FOR CORROSIVE POISONS!**

Activated Charcoal

After first-aid suggestions for noncorrosive poisons have been followed and medical help is delayed due to travel or other reasons, activated charcoal may be administered to hopefully absorb the remaining poison. It does not absorb all poisons and a rather large amount may be required for it to be effective. For example: it takes 1-1/2 ounces of charcoal powder (about 10 grams) to bind 3 adult aspirin. Mix the charcoal with water into a thick soup for the victim to drink.

HERBAL AIDES:

Milk Thistle: Milk Thistle is known around the world as one of the best natural aids for protecting and healing the liver. It is best known for it's ability to cure the Death cap mushroom poison. According to David Hoffmann, he suggests that the best results with using Milk thistle are found in toxic metabolic hepatitis and cirrhosis, in that it shortens the length of viral hepatitis, minimizes complications and also protects the liver against problems arising from surgery. He writes, "This all goes to make it an excellent remedy to use in the prevention and treatments of many liver disorders. The earlier treatment is commenced the better the prognosis but effective treatment is possible at virtually every stage."

DOSAGE: Milk thistle can be taken in the powdered form, also as an infusion, a decoction, glycerine extract, and also alcohol extract, with the alcohol extract being the strongest.

In the powdered form a dosage of two to four grams three times per day is normal. For the infusion use one teaspoonful of the powdered herb to 150 ml of boiling distilled water left to infuse for ten minutes and drink this three times per day. For the decoction use three teaspoonfuls of the seeds to half a pint of distilled water and simmer for about twenty minutes, drink this three times per day. In the case of the glycerine and alcohol extract take 2.5 mls three times per day. In the case of poisoning where there is need to act quickly take 1:1 liquid extract at doses of 10 mls three or more times per day.

In severe poising cases, I would use a dropperfull every hour for 8 to 10 hours.

Dr. Christopher's Liver and Gallbladder Formula: This is a tried and true formula we have used in the clinic for over 20 years. It helps tone and cleanse the liver. It is best used in conjunction with other holistic aids during poisoning, though we have seen it effective when we had nothing else to use. On one occasion, our cat had eaten a poisonous animal such as a toad. He was almost dead when we found him, lethargic and barely breathing. He would take no water and could not lift his head and was quite limp. We used an eyedropper and gave him water and the Liver and Gallbladder Formula.

In this case we gave him an eyedropper full every half an hour. All together it took about two hours but eventually he started to move around and was able to get up and quickly gained a full recovery.

The formula is

3 parts Barberry (Berberis vulgaris)

1 part Wild yam (Dioscorea villosa)

1 part Cramp bark (Viburnum trilobum)

1 part Fennel seed (Foeniculum vulgare)

1 part Ginger (Zingiber officinalis)

1 part Catnip (Nepeta cataria)

1 part Peppermint (Mentha piperita)

Plantain (Plantago major): It has been used historically as an excellent aid against such poisons as snake bit and black widow. Plantain is also used as an antivenomous herb in its role as a blood cleanser. Terry Willard, author of *Edible and Medicinal Plants of the Rocky Mountains and Neighbouring Territories*, states that it is good to draw out the poison of snake bites. It is an excellent choice for poisonous bites and stings of scorpions and insects.

Plantain is #1 in the field of blood poisoning treatment. You can see the healing at work. Swelling goes down and the "red" line recedes. Limbs poisoned can be saved using this herb. It is used as a poultice on the outside and taken as a tea on the inside.

It is best in this case to take as a tincture or a tea orally to get it into the system quickly. The tea is made with one teaspoon to a cup of water or a tablespoon to a pint. Drink at least five cups a day during an episode of poising. It the poison is from a bite or a sting, then also put a poultice of plantain on the wound to aid in drawing out the poison.

An incident that occurred with me several years was helped greatly from this plant. I had been bitten on the hand by a spider and it became a nasty looking ulcer and infected. I made a poultice of the fresh leaves (can be found in most yards that haven't had all of the "weeds" removed) and left it on over night. Very quickly I noticed the pain diminishing. By morning, I removed the poultice and the infection had been completely drawn out the wound was sealing. A truly amazing wonder of a plant, and considered such a "weed" by so many.

Dr. Christopher's Blood Stream Formula: According to Dr. Christopher, the Blood Purifying Formula containing red clover, chaparral, licorice root, poke root, peach bark, Oregon grape root, stillingia, prickly ash bark, burdock root, and buckthorn bark. This formula creates, not only a generalized blood purifier, but also includes a group of herbs that aid in building strength and cleaning out the entire body, by helping break loose toxic deposits and flush them out, and also acting as a food for the organs.

DOSAGE: During a poisoning event this formula, used in conjunction with any of the above methods will aid in speeding up the healing process by getting the poisons out of the blood more quickly. During a crisis, I would use one dropperful every hour for six to eight hours, until the crisis has passed.

The formula:

2 parts Red Clover blossoms (Trifolium pratense)

1 part Chaparral (Larrea tridentata)

1 part Licorice root (Glycyrrhiza glabra)

1 part Poke root (Phytolacca americana)

1 part Peach bark (Prunus persica)

1 part Oregon grape root (Mahonia aquifolium)

1 part Stillingia (Stillingia sylvatica)

1 part Cascara sagrada (Rhamnus purshiana)

1 part Sarsaparilla (Smilax aspera)

1 part Prickly ash bark (Zanthoxylum americanum)

1 part Burdock root (Arctium lappa)

1 part Buckthorn bark (Rhamnus frangula)

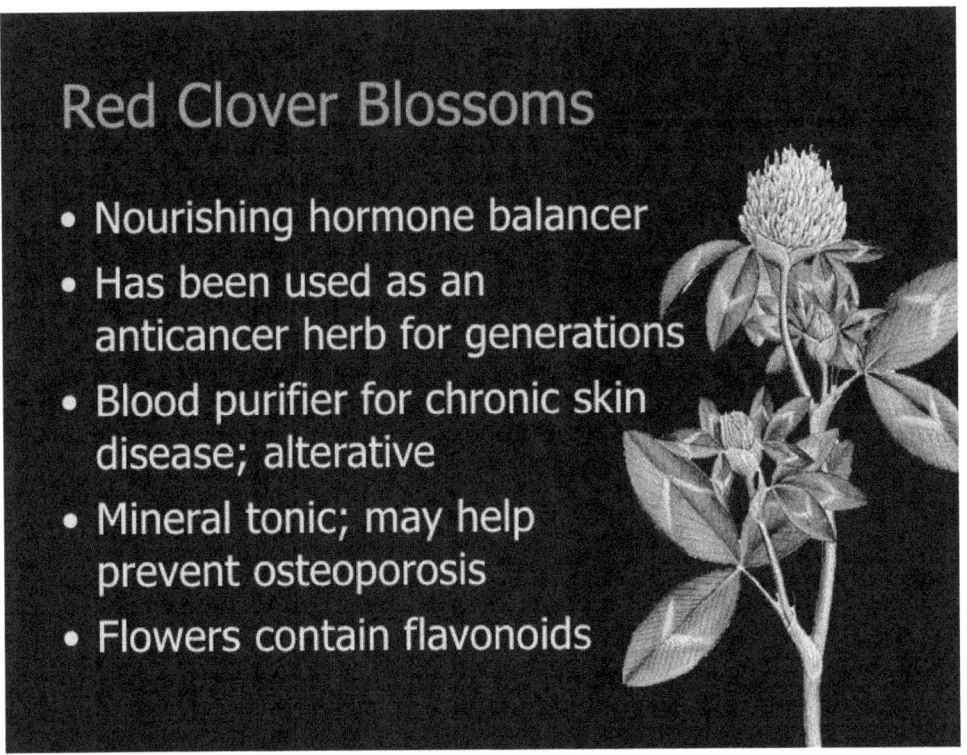

Red Clover Blossoms

- Nourishing hormone balancer
- Has been used as an anticancer herb for generations
- Blood purifier for chronic skin disease; alterative
- Mineral tonic; may help prevent osteoporosis
- Flowers contain flavonoids

4.3 Broken bones

Broken bones rank towards the top of some of the most painful and serious emergencies you may encounter and one of the scariest without a qualified healthcare provider present. It can be from simple fall off a chair to hiking though the mountains with no one around. This is again one of the those situations where it is often best to get to a hospital but we will cover what you can do without such access. We will also discuss what you can do if you have received emergency room treatment and would like to heal faster.

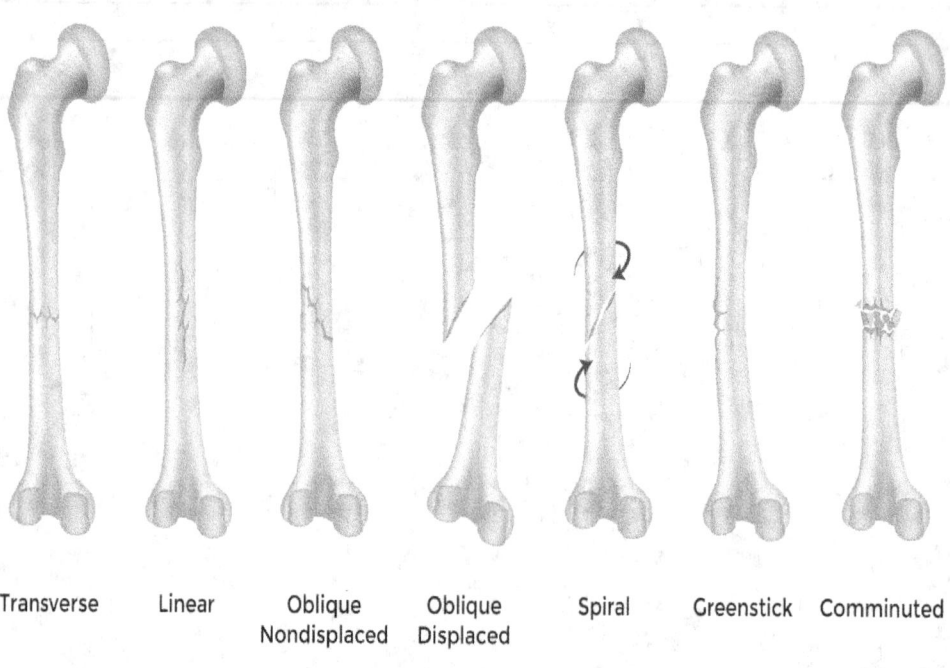

Transverse   Linear   Oblique Nondisplaced   Oblique Displaced   Spiral   Greenstick   Comminuted

Types of broken bones

BASIC BROKEN BONE FIRST AID:

According to the Mayo clinic:

A fracture is a broken bone. It requires medical attention. If the broken bone is the result of major trauma or injury, call 911 or your local emergency number.
Also call for emergency help if:

- The person is unresponsive, isn't breathing or isn't moving. Begin CPR if there's no breathing or heartbeat.
- There is heavy bleeding.
- Even gentle pressure or movement causes pain.
- The limb or joint appears deformed.
- The bone has pierced the skin.
- The extremity of the injured arm or leg, such as a toe or finger, is numb or bluish at the tip.
- You suspect a bone is broken in the neck, head or back.

Don't move the person except if necessary to avoid further injury. Take these actions immediately while waiting for medical help:

- **Stop any bleeding.** Apply pressure to the wound with a sterile bandage, a clean cloth or a clean piece of clothing.
- **Immobilize the injured area.** Don't try to realign the bone or push a bone that's sticking out back in. If you've been trained in how to splint and professional help isn't readily available, apply a splint to the area above and below the fracture sites. Padding the splints can help reduce discomfort.
- **Apply ice packs to limit swelling and help relieve pain.** Don't apply ice directly to the skin. Wrap the ice in a towel, piece of cloth or some other material.
- **Treat for shock.** If the person feels faint or is breathing in short, rapid breaths, lay the person down with the head slightly lower than the trunk and, if possible, elevate the legs. We discussed this in the section on Bleeding.

HERBAL AIDS:

Dr. Christopher's B, F and C Formula: This is by far the best formula I have used for encouraging rapid healing of a broken bone. As stated earlier; B, F and C stands for Bone, Flesh and Cartilage. The formula is described in the section **Major Bleeding/Shock/Deep Cuts and Wounds.**

Dr. Christopher often recommended a calcium tea with Comfrey to help with mending broken bones. An example was:

Comfrey Tea and Organic Calcium: After the doctor has set the bone, drink three or more cups of Comfrey tea each day--the more the better. With each cup of tea take the calcium combination. This is the formula:

6 parts Horsetail grass
4 parts Comfrey root
3 parts Oat straw
1 part Lobelia

For children old enough to take capsules, use two capsules or more, three times in a day. As suggested, take these capsules with the Comfrey tea. Mix the powder with blackstrap molasses, if it is hard to swallow the capsules.

Broken Bones After Being Set: After a doctor has set the bone, drink three or more cups of Complete Tissue & Bone and/or Comfrey tea or green drink per day. With each cup take two or more capsules of the Calc formula.

Here was a testimonial given to Dr. Christopher quite a few years ago: *"Over the years of practice I have had a number of patients who have had broken bones from osteoporosis. One case was a woman in her middle eighties with a fractured hip. After three months in a cast it showed no sign of healing, any more than two pieces of stick growing together. This woman was frightened because she was told that if the hip bones did not knit after putting on another cast for three months, they would cut her leg open and use stainless steel rods, bolts and nuts to make it possible for her to at least get around on crutches. This was in the early sixties and not much Comfrey was available then. The lady's daughter was in one of my classes, and we asked the students to help out by donating as much Comfrey as they could. We had enough donated from the class members that the patient had from a pint to a quart of Comfrey green drink or Comfrey tea each day, six days a week, week after week. At the end of this "three months," the cast was removed and the doctors were amazed, because during the first three months were was "no knitting" of the bone even evident, but with the Comfrey being taken orally during the next three-month period the leg was healed. The daughter told us her mother was out square dancing within a couple of weeks after the cast was removed!*

Since this case was so outstanding we have had a formula developed called "bone, flesh and cartilage."[Complete Tissue & Bone] This formula has done miraculous things with broken backs, legs, hips, etc. This formula has been used to help with curvature of the spine, polio, multiple sclerosis, and muscular dystrophy, stroke and arthritis of the bone. This formula is used externally as well as orally and has brought tremendously fast results."

If taken as capsules for mending a broken bone I have found that 3 capsules 4 times day works well and for a more rapid healing I would use 5 capsules 5 times a day. I have seen broken bones healed in a third to half of the time usually seen in conventional medicine.

Comfrey: If you do not have access to the above formulas then Comfrey alone can do the job. It has a history of thousands of years in promoting bone health when a fracture has occurred. It can be made as a poultice, a fomentation, taken as a tea or in capsule form.

The roots are more potent than the leaves but if you cannot get them than the leaves will help:

Decoction 2 fluid ounces three times daily.
Fluid extract ½-2 teaspoonfuls.
Infusion 1 cupful, 3 times daily.
Powder 2 #00 capsules or 1 teaspoonful
Tincture ½-1 teaspoonful (fluid teaspoon)

4.4 Heart Attack/Strokes

HEART ATTACK FACTS:

According to the CDC; **every 40 seconds**, someone in the United States has a heart attack.

A heart attack, also called a myocardial infarction, occurs when a part of the heart muscle doesn't receive enough blood flow. The more time that passes without treatment to restore blood flow, the greater the damage to the heart muscle.

Every year, about **790,000 Americans** have a heart attack. Of these cases

- 580,000 are a first heart attack.
- 210,000 happen to people who have already had a first heart attack.[1]

One of 5 heart attacks is silent—the damage is done, but the person is not aware of it.

The five major symptoms of a heart attack are

- Pain or discomfort in the jaw, neck, or back.
- Feeling weak, light-headed, or faint.
- Chest pain or discomfort.
- Pain or discomfort in arms or shoulder.
- Shortness of breath.

Other symptoms of a heart attack could include unusual or unexplained tiredness and nausea or vomiting. Women are more likely to have these other symptoms.

STROKE FACTS:

Stroke is the fifth leading cause of death in the United States and is a major cause of serious disability for adults. About **795,000** people in the United States have a stroke each year.

Stroke Statistics

- Stroke kills about **140,000** Americans each year—that's **1 out of every 20 deaths**.
- Someone in the United States has a stroke every **40 seconds**. Every **4 minutes**, someone dies of stroke.
- Every year, more than **795,000 people** in the United States have a stroke. About 610,000 of these are first or new strokes.
- About 185,000 strokes—**nearly 1 of 4**—are in people who have had a previous stroke.
- About **87%** of all strokes are ischemic strokes, in which blood flow to the brain is blocked.
- Stroke costs the United States an estimated **$34 billion** each year. This total includes the cost of health care services, medicines to treat stroke, and missed days of work.
- Stroke is a leading cause of serious long-term disability. Stroke reduces mobility in more than half of stroke survivors age 65 and over.

Unfortunately, the average person is completely unaware that they are even at risk so they are caught by surprise when it happens. In most cases, this means they are completely unprepared. What can we do for ourselves and our family members to help them have more than the "four golden minutes" needed to save their lives in the event of a heart attack or stroke?

As stated before, we return to our favorite herb for emergencies … Cayenne! Not too surprised are you after reading this whole book? There is NO better herb that can be used for this issues than capsicum annum (cayenne).

We discussed this in some detail earlier but I will detail a few more facts and what you can do in an emergency.

A common protocol recommended by Dr. Christopher and one I have used in my practice is as follows:

Heart Attack: Prop up the patient and pour hot cayenne tea down, (use a teaspoonful of cayenne in a cup of hot water), and have the patient drink the full cup. and the attack will stop immediately. We have been called in the middle of the night so many times. A teaspoon of cayenne should bring the patient out of the heart attack. In case cayenne is not around and you have a heart attack, the dosage on black pepper can be tripled and used.

I have personally seen this technique work and save lives. It will also work on a stroke victim if you get them to take it. If not, I have seen where you can get cayenne tincture or the water with cayenne in it, in an eyedropper (plastic so they don't bite down on it and hurt themselves) and place it on their tongue. The reaction is pretty quick and it can save lives.

As mentioned before, this is due to the fact that cayenne can cause an equalization of blood pressure throughout the body momentarily which in turn takes the pressure off the heart or brain.

Please consider always having a bottle of cayenne tincture available for emergencies. As a tincture it can last for many, many years stored in a cool, dark place such as a medicine cabinet, a purse, etc.

Hawthorne berry Syrup: This is a great herb which has been used historically for heart and circulatory repair. It has been used for thousands of years for such issues as Congestive Heart Failure, arrhythmia, etc. But it also can work on a heart attack. A testimonial given to Dr. Christopher stated:

"One doctor who had learned the formula for Hawthorn berry syrup from Dr. Christopher raised his hand after a lecture to tell the following story. He had gone on a house call in response to a call about a heart attack, one so serious that the family was afraid that death was imminent. The doctor had no cayenne in his bag and the family had no cayenne; the doctor began to panic. He remembered that he had a bottle of Hawthorn berry syrup with him. The usual dose is a half-teaspoonful, but the doctor thought a little more might help, so he gave the patient a full tablespoonful. The patient drank it down, sat right up, and said, "Well, I feel okay". The doctor checked him with the stethoscope and the heart sounded alright. As the doctor said, "Talk about quick relief!"

STOP HEART ATTACK WITH CAYENNE PEPPER

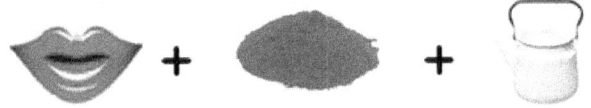

CAYENNE PEPPER   HOT WATER

Dr. John Christopher: *"In 35 years of practice I have never on house calls lost one heart attack patient. The reason is if they are still breathing -- I pour 1 tsp of cayenne in a cup of hot water, and within minutes they are up and around."*

NOTE:
First the Cayenne pepper must be at least 90,000 heat units or 90,000(H.U) to be able to stop a heart.

• If the cayenne is at least 90,000 H.U. and the person is still conscious, the recommendation is to mix 1 tsp of cayenne powder in a glass of warm water, and give it to the person to drink.

• If the person is unconscious then the recommendation is to use a cayenne extract (at least 90,000 H.U), and put 2 full droppers underneath their tongue.

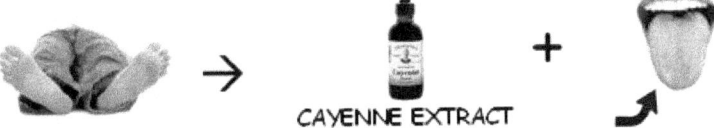

CAYENNE EXTRACT

facebook.com/stepintomygreenworld   pinterest.com/mygreenworld

4.5 Pain Management

One of the most important aspects of treating a patient in an emergency situation is pain management. Without this it can often be difficult to care for an injured patient when they are not able to relax and give in to the care. It can also lead a patient further into shock.

Within the holistic, natural world, most of the best pain killers are illegal so we have to make do with what is available to us. The good news is that there are some very good options for relieving pain.

HERBAL AIDS:

Bugleweed (Lycopus virginicus):

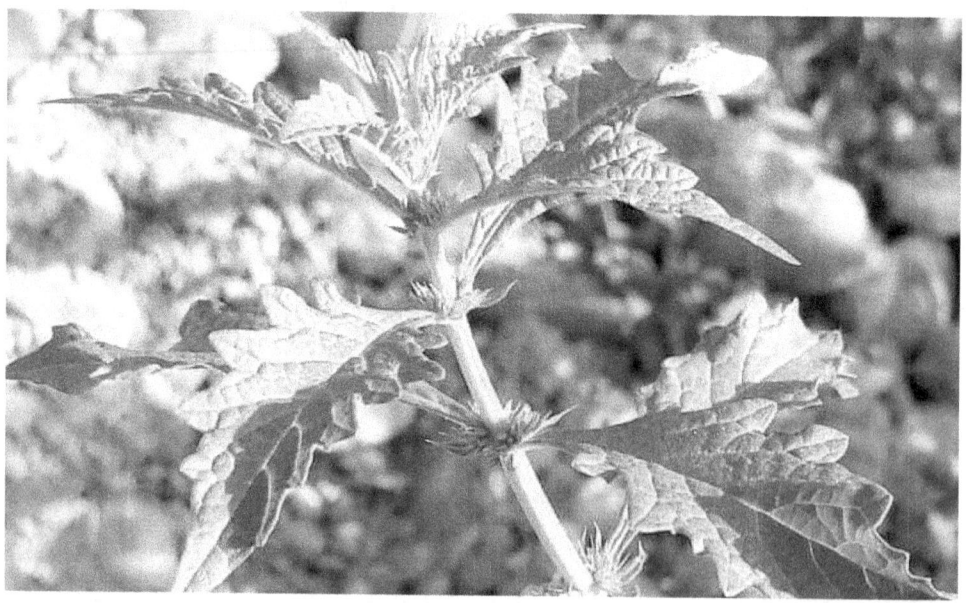

Known botanically as *Lycopus virginicus*, this is a perennial plant that generally thrives in damp regions. The herb actually belongs to the mint family but lacks the familiar minty odor of real mint. Some of its most common uses include treating respiratory illness and bringing balance to the hormones. It's use in this case is it's ability to be slight narcotic. It can be used as a great pain reliever.

I have a personal story with Bugleweed. Many years ago I was scheduled to have all of my wisdom teeth removed along with a cyst that had been caused by the pressure of one of the teeth. Knowing that I would not use any of the pain killers that would be prescribed for post-surgery I made up a pot of the tea the night before.

After my wife got me home and put me to bed she brought in a cup of the tea. I must tell you that the tea has a very strong flavor and will most likely be unpleasant to most people. I personally did not care. I drank the tea and laid back to relax. After about twenty minutes my wife came back to check on me to see if I was in any pain. The mild narcotic properties of the tea not only kept the pain away but made me very happy with a tendency to giggle. For the next few days all I used for a pain killer was a cup of the tea two or three times a day for a few days. I also healed very quickly with no dry sockets from the removal.

It can also be used as a tincture or in capsule form.

DOSAGE: As a tea: 1 cup full as needed for pain. As capsules two to three capsules as needed. As a tincture 2 to four dropperfuls as needed for pain.

Cramp bark and Valerian:

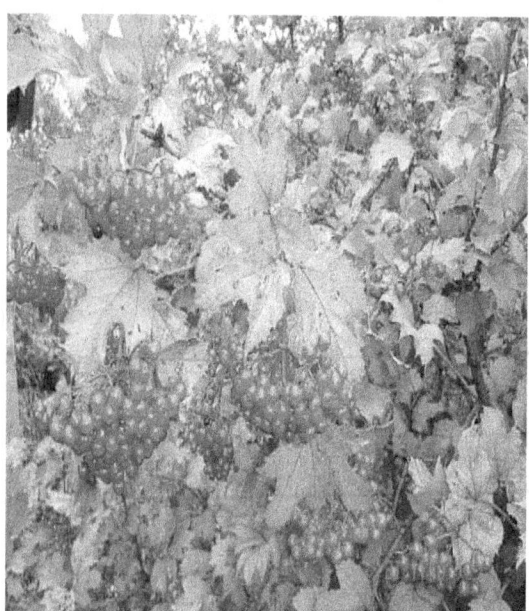 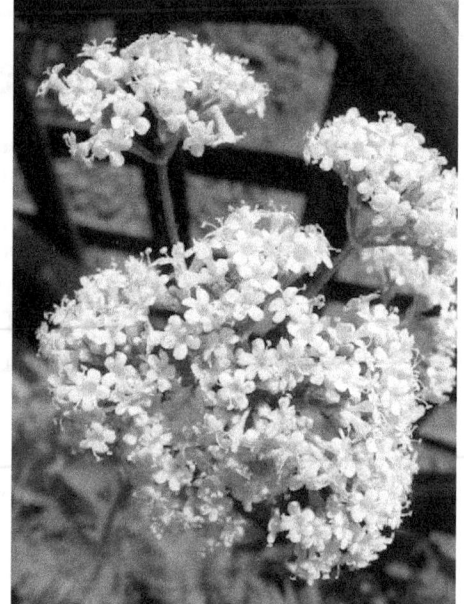

Crampbark and Valerian

This is a wonderful combination we have put together as a mixture of a muscle relaxer and a pain killer. **Cramp bark** (Viburnum opulus) has been used historically by the Native Americans for hundreds of years as a muscle relaxer, especially by women for menstrual cramps. I sprained my back years ago and it was a very effective muscle relaxer.

Valerian (Valeriana officinalis) is well known in the holistic community for it's superb ability for killing pain and for its effect as a tranquilizer and nervine, particularly for those people suffering from nervous over strain. Valerian has been shown to encourage sleep, improve sleep quality and reduce blood pressure. It is also used internally in the treatment of painful menstruation, cramps, hypertension, irritable bowel syndrome etc.

The two herbs are best used as a tincture for faster action. We combine an equal amount of each herb and make an alcohol based tincture from it.

DOSAGE: For adults we usually recommend 1 to 2 dropperfuls as needed for pain. You can increase the dosage easily to four dropperfuls as needed but be aware that the higher the dosage the more relaxed you can become and the "loopier". It may not be safe to drive or operate machinery at higher doses.

Willow (Salix alba):

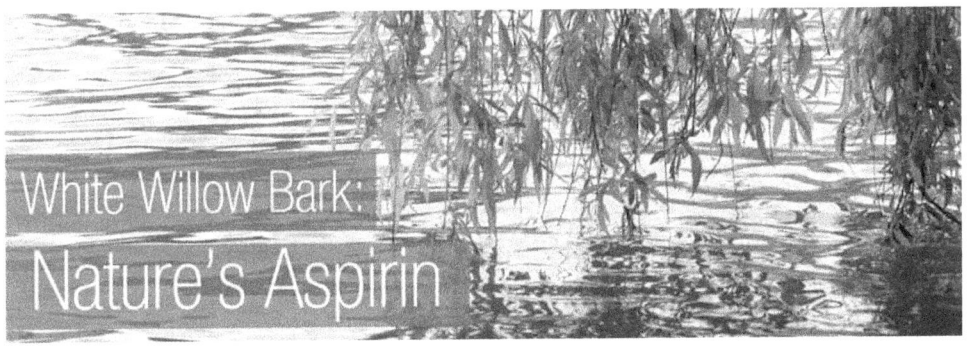

As the picture indicates .. the original source for aspirin. The year was 1899 and Bayer came out with Bayer aspirin. They knew they could not patent a Popular or Willow tree so the worked on extracting what they considered the key ingredient from the plant for relieving pain ... salicin. After purifying it they produced salicylic acid .. aspirin. There was a problem with this extraction though. Left in the original Willow or Poplar bark it is suspended and buffered by hundreds of other chemical constituents. In it's form as aspirin it is not buffered by nature and can eat a hole in your stomach. Not so with Willow.

DOSAGE: We have used it as a tea, capsule or as a tincture. Again, the tincture and tea form are faster acting. The capsule form takes longer to take effect but lasts longer. It is very safe. Use two capsules or dropperfuls or a cup of tea as needed for pain.

CBD:

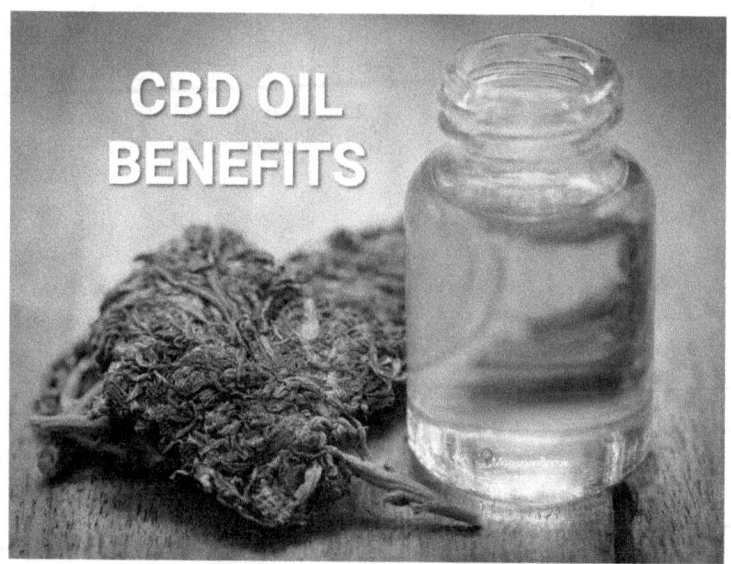

Praised by many and reviled by others, there seems to very little middle ground for the acceptance of this natural remedy. Yes, it does come from Cannabis but we are talking about the form with no THC in it. It does not have any narcotic effects.

We have used it for many years and seen patients who could not take a pharmaceutical drug find relief. Be careful of your supplier of CBD products. Since legalization in many states vendors have come out of the wood work. We prefer to use a company called CV Sciences. They seem to be very consistent in their quality. They are out of Colorado.

DOSAGE: CBD can come in MANY forms. You can get it as capsules, as an oil, salves, sprays, etc. We use it mainly in capsule and salve form. For most folks, they can take one to two of the capsules as needed for pain or to aid in sleeping as needed. The salve is wonderful as a topical application for pain, such as muscle aches.

Castor Oil Packs:

Castor oil packs are age old in their history and are as good today as when they were used hundreds of years ago. The concept is actually quite simple. You take a clean, white cotton cloth and soak in castor oil and place it over the area that is in pain. Cover it with a piece of saran wrap and then a towel. Over the towel you place a heating pad. That's it.

It is able to relieve pain through the use of the castor oil soaking into the skin and getting both the blood and the lymphatic circulation moving. It becomes very cleansing in action and can relieve pain in a matter of minutes.

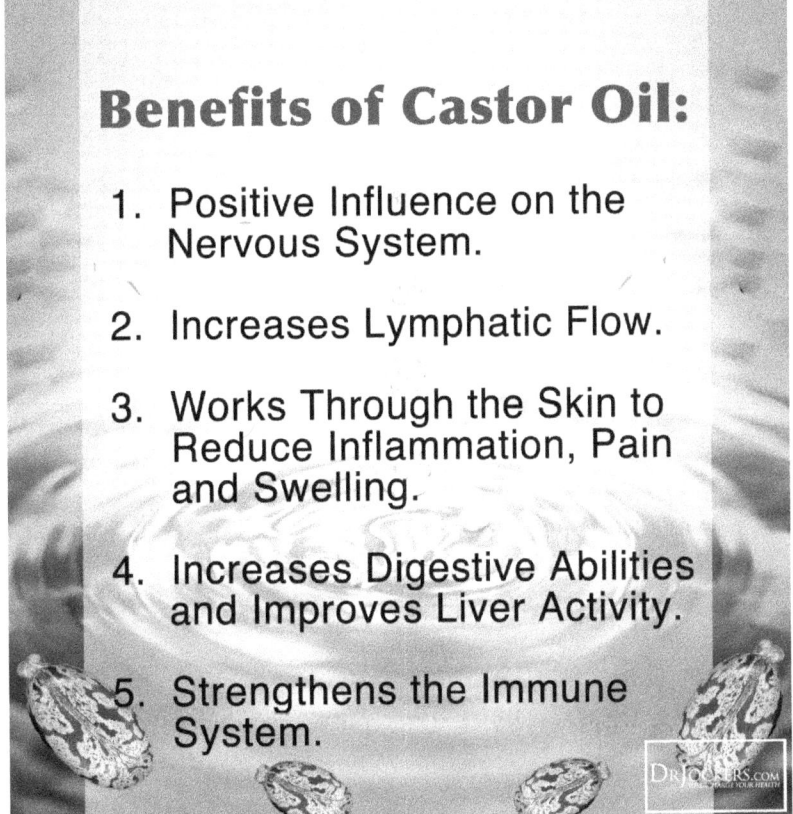

Cayenne Deep Heating:

In an earlier section of this book I discussed Cayenne's ability to be a Rubefacient. This is defined as an herb which can cause a gentle and localized increase in the surface blood flow. This brings along with it more oxygen and nutrients. This will make the area appear red due to the increased blood flow. All of this aids in the healing process which helps diminish pain.

It is well known that a deep heating salve soothes painful and tired muscles. Rather than make our own we generally use Dr. Christopher's Heat ointment.

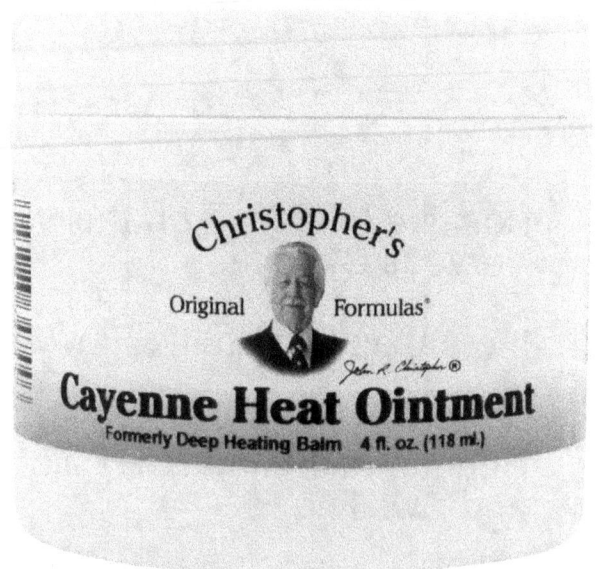

Dr. Christoper's Heat Ointment

Ingredients: Cayenne Pepper (40,000 H.U.), Virgin Olive Oil, Oil of Wintergreen, Menthol Crystals & other pure essential oils as fragrances & Beeswax.

Cold/Hot Packs:

Finally, an oldie but goodie, cold and hot packs. Applying ice or heat can provide relief from injuries, aches, and pains. Ice works for injuries because it narrows your blood vessels, which helps prevent blood from accumulating at the site of injury, which will add to inflammation and swelling while delaying healing. This is also why elevation is helpful, since it limits blood flow to the area to minimize swelling.

For muscle aches and pains, applying a heat pack will help bring blood flow to the area, which promotes healing and soothes pain while increasing flexibility. As blood flow increases, so does the flow of oxygen and nutrients to the area while waste materials are removed. Heat also works well for joint pain or as a pre-workout warm-up. Hot gel packs or heated water bottles work well for this

They are very simple to use and we have seen patients receive great relief from them. The general rule of thumb is to switch them out as each has their own benefits. Initially, place a hot pack on the patient for 12 minutes. The switch to a cold pack for 4 minutes. switch back and forth for as long as the patient feels comfortable doing so. Make sure to have a towel laid down first over the area and then place the packs on top of it.

I have seen cases of appendicitis clear up with the aid of the hot and cold packs being done all night over the area of the appendix. It can also help get the bowels moving during stubborn cases of constipation or a bowel blockage when done over the abdominal region.

HOW TO MAKE THE HOT PACK:
This can be as simple as a hot water bottle or an electric heating pad (some do not care for the EMF coming off of it) or you can fill a sock with rice, sew up the end and heat it in the microwave.

HOW TO MAKE THE COLD PACK:
Again, very simple. Many folks just file a zip-lock bag full of ice.

CHAPTER 5
A SAMPLE FIRST-AID KIT

I would like to take some time now to help you figure out how to make your own Holistic, First Aid kit. In this section we will discuss where to buy them or if you choose to, how to make your own from scratch.

5.1   First Aid Kit Supplies

As far as Dr. Christopher's products are concerned, they can be purchased at Dr. Christoper's Herb Shop online. The website is **https://www.drchristophersherbshop.com**. I will place a * next to the product in the kit if it can be purchased from them or another online source.

Below is a list of what we would put into a home, holistic first aid kit. Please feel free to modify this for your own needs.

FIRST AID KIT SUPPLIES:

For pain relief:
*CBD oil/salve or capsules – CV Sciences 855-758-7223
Cramp bark and Valerian Tincture.
*Willow tincture or capsules – Dr. Christopher's Herb Shop. - 801-489-4500
*Cayenne Heat Ointment - Dr. Christopher's Herb Shop. - 801-489-4500
Aloe Vera gel.

For treating and preventing infection:
Herbadyne
*Garlic oil - Dr. Christopher's Herb Shop. - 801-489-4500
*Infection Formula - Dr. Christopher's Herb Shop. - 801-489-4500

Eye Injuries:
*Herbal Eyebright - Dr. Christopher's Herb Shop. - 801-489-4500

For wound healing:

Green Salve
Comfrey paste ingredients.
*Comfrey root powder - Dr. Christopher's Herb Shop. - 801-489-4500
Raw honey
*Wheatgerm oil - Dr. Christopher's Herb Shop. - 801-489-4500
*Dr. Christopher's Ear and Nerve - Dr. Christopher's Herb Shop. - 801-489-4500
*Dr. Christopher's Complete Tissue and Bone (B, F and C) capsules and salve. Dr. Christopher's Herb Shop. - 801-489-4500

For bleeding/heart attack/strokes/shock:
*Cayenne Tincture - Dr. Christopher's Herb Shop. - 801-489-4500

For poisoning:
*Plantain Tincture - Dr. Christopher's Herb Shop. - 801-489-4500
Activated charcoal

For nausea:
Ginger – As an herb for tea or capsules or drink.

For allergies and allergy related shock:
*Dr. Christopher's Kid-e-Soothe - Dr. Christopher's Herb Shop. - 801-489-4500
*Stinging Nettle tincture – The herb itself can be bought at - Dr. Christopher's Herb Shop. - 801-489-4500. The you can make your own tincture.

Magnifying glass for checking out splinters, ticks, etc.
Tick remover.
Bandages of various sizes.
Gauze pads of various sizes.
Hot water bottle or a heating pad.
Cold pack ready made or a zip-lock bag.
Pack of butterfly bandages.
Ace bandages.
Finger splint.
1 adhesive cloth tape (10 yards x 1 inch)
2 absorbent compress dressings (5 x 9 inches)

Tweezers
2 pairs of non-latex gloves.
Clean cotton cloth.
Bulb syringe.

5.2 How to make your own medications

While it may be convenient to purchase your holistic medications, I feel it is important that we each know how to make our own in a pinch. You can also save a LOT of money should you decide to make your own.

Several of these instructions have already been detailed in this book but I wanted to give you an easy look up for them in one place.

Making a tincture:
The rule of thumb for most tinctures uses a 4:1 ratio of the medium to the herbs. The medium is usually 100 proof vodka as it is 50% water and 50% alcohol. This is the best of both worlds as some herbs require water and some alcohol to be extracted.

For example, if you are going to have 8 ounces of alcohol than you would use 2 ounces of herbs. The herbs can be cut or powdered but powdered can be harder to filter out later in the process.

Place the herbs in the jar and pour in the vodka. Seal and write on it the date you started it. Shake well.

Store in a cool, dark place for two weeks, making sure to walk by at least once a day and shake vigorously.

Drain the tincture though cheesecloth to remove the herbs from the liquid.

Pour the strained tincture into smaller, colored bottles and cap. Be sure to label the bottles. The tincture will keep indefinitely in a cool area.

This formula works well on most herbs, certainly all of those mentioned in this book, including Stinging nettle, Cayenne, Plantain and such.

Making a fomentation:

A fomentation is a cloth soaked in a strong tea and placed over the area of concern. Make a tea out of the herb using 1 teaspoon of the herb to a cup of distilled water or a tablespoon to a pint. Boil the water and not the herb. Let the water boil and when rolling, take off the burner and put the herb in the water, cover and let steep for 20 to 25 minutes or more. Soak the white cotton cloth in it and then place over the area. Cover with saran wrap to keep the moisture and heat in. Leave on for 25 minutes and repeat as often during the day as needed.

Making a Poultice:

A poultice is a wrap made from the actual plant material. Take the plant and tear or break up and put in a pan with distilled water. Put on low simmer for about 25 to 30 minutes. Take the plant materiel out along with some of the water and place on a piece of white, cotton cloth or flannel. Wrap the affected area with the plant in direct contact with the skin and wrap an ace bandage on it to keep it in place. It can be kept on overnight and changed the next day as needed.

Making an infusion (a tea):

An infusion is simply a tea from the flowers, leaves or stems of a plant. Make a tea out of the herb using 1 teaspoon of the herb to a cup of distilled water or a tablespoon to a pint. Boil the water and not the herb. Let the water boil and when rolling, take off the burner and put the herb in the water, cover and let steep for 20 to 25 minutes or more.

Making onion cough syrup:

Take white or yellow onion and chop it up and place into a sauce pan. Cover with raw honey and simmer over low heat for about 25 to 30 minutes. Strain and use the honey as a teaspoon to a tablespoon as needed for coughs.

Making an onion poultice:

To make the poultice, take a white or yellow onion and chop it up thoroughly. Place in the oven at about 250 to 300 degrees for about twenty minutes. You will know when it is done as the pieces are just starting to get "slimy". Now take them out and let them cool enough where they will not damage the skin and place over the chest while the patient is lying down. If this is for a baby then please make sure to rub some olive oil on the skin first to protect it as they are more sensitive than older children or adults.

Making a castor oil pack:

To do this soak a white cotton cloth in castor oil and place it over the skin of the area affected. Now cover the cloth with a saran wrap and then place a towel over the wrap. Now place a heating pad over the towel Do this as many times a day as you can, at least twice a day.

Making an Herbadyne tincture:

Ingredients are 2 ounces of powdered Myrrh, one ounce powdered Golden seal, ½ ounce of powdered cayenne and one quart of 100 proof vodka.

Combine all of the herbs and alcohol in a glass jar, cap tightly and keep it in a cool, shaded area for 14 days. Shake at least once each day. Strain and keep the alcohol in a dark bottle and store in a cool place.

Making a salve:

While this is actually pretty easy, it can take a little practice getting the correct amount of bees wax at the end. Too little and the salve is watery and too much and you might as well be using a rock. Let's give this a try.

You will need the following ingredients:

The herb (Lets try Chickweed for now as a nice skin soother)
Cold pressed, extra virgin, organic Olive oil.
Beeswax.

Place the cut up herb (Chickweed for example) in the pan and cover about an inch over with the Olive oil. Turn the heat on low and let simmer for about 20 minutes. Cover. Try not to let it boil. Check now and then.

After about twenty minutes turn off the heat and move the pan to a burner that is off and cool. Let sit with the cover on it for about 1 hour or more, until it has cooled enough for you to be able to safely strain it. Then strain the oil through a white, cotton cloth or cheese cloth into a bowl.

Clean the previous pan and then put the oil back into it. Turn the heat on to a low setting, careful not to boil. You will need to frequently stir so as not to burn the oil. When the oil is hot, being to CAREFULLY add a little bit of bees wax to the oil and let it melt. Now comes the tricky part. You need to test each time to make sure if you have enough bees wax in the mixture.

To test it, have ready a little saucer or cup with some water in it. Take a little spoonful of the oil and drop into the water. If it remains an oil after cooling than add more bees wax to the hot oil. If it turns to wax then you are done!

Before it has completely cooled, pour in jars and place in the fridge to store. You want it in the fridge relatively soon or it may start to separate. Your done. In a cool, dark place it can last a year at a good potency.

About The Author

Dr. Earendil M. Spindelilus D.N.M., M.H., C.R. - Traditional Naturopath, Holistic Practitioner, Clinical Master Herbalist, Certified Nutritionist, Certified Reflexology, Member of Plant Savers of America, Member of American Botanical Council.

I hold a Doctorate degree in Natural Medicine. I have also been a lecturer since 1999. Board Certified Diplomate of Natural Medicine. Member of the American Council of Holistic Medicine.

I have always had a deep and abiding interest in the Plant Kingdom. Even very young I loved the way the herbs held the mystery of healing within them and how I could learn about them. I traveled around the world learning from different cultures their own unique floras and how they incorporated them into their daily lives. With each new herb I learned how special the world is and how Nature supplies us with all we need. In the 1990s I decided to take my education further and enrolled in the School and Natural Healing, the College of Herbal Medicine. I graduated in 1999 with my Master Herbalist. I have also studied with the New Eden School of Natural Medicine where I completed my Doctorate in Natural Medicine. To date, my wife and I have run two medical centers for natural healing. It has always been a great joy meeting with our patients. We are all meant to live a happy, healthy life and when we allow the body to perform it's innate ability to heal itself then this can happen. I am also a past board member of the Reflexology Association of California as well as a published author/writer of numerous holistic books and articles. I am also a past host of a holistic radio show.

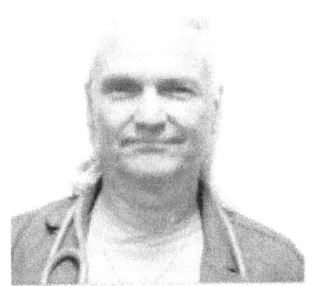

www.ingramcontent.com/pod-product-compliance
Lightning Source LLC
Chambersburg PA
CBHW070605220526
45467CB00003B/1314